听妈妈讲中药故事

（双语手绘版）

Mama's Storytelling of Chinese Medicine

（ *Bilingual hand-painted version* ）

主 编　陈 华　齐昌菊　郁东海

Editor　Chen Hua　Qi Changju　Yu Donghai

中医古籍出版社

图书在版编目（CIP）数据

听妈妈讲中药故事：双语手绘版 / 陈华，齐昌菊，郁东海主编 . —北京：中医古籍出版社，2018.7
ISBN 978-7-5152-1672-0

Ⅰ. ①听…　Ⅱ. ①陈…②齐…③郁…　Ⅲ. ①中草药 – 儿童读物　Ⅳ. ① R282–49

中国版本图书馆 CIP 数据核字（2018）第 029004 号

听妈妈讲中药故事（双语手绘版）

主编　陈　华　齐昌菊　郁东海

责任编辑　贾萧荣
封面设计　李　绮　赵石涛
漫画绘图　程钰涵　李　琦
排版设计　李　绮
出版发行　中医古籍出版社
社　　址　北京东直门内南小街 16 号（100700）
电　　话　010-64089446（总编室）010-64002949（发行部）
网　　址　www.zhongyiguji.com.cn
印　　刷　北京博海升彩色印刷有限公司
开　　本　880mm×1230mm　1/16
印　　张　6.5
字　　数　120 千字
版　　次　2018 年 7 月第 1 版　2018 年 7 月第 1 次印刷
书　　号　ISBN 978-7-5152-1672-0
定　　价　42.00 元

编 委 会

前 言

2017 年 7 月 1 日，《中华人民共和国中医药法》正式实施，支持和鼓励中医药科普，指出应"加强中医药文化宣传，普及中医药知识，鼓励组织和个人创作中医药文化和科普作品"。

传统的中医药科普图书因为词汇生涩、语句深奥，很难被小朋友们理解，如何打破这些阻碍中医药知识传播的障碍，是摆在中医科普从业者面前的一道难题。

基于以上思考，我们选择了用生动鲜活的手绘漫画来传递古老的中医药文化知识的精髓，让生涩深奥的理论知识变成浅显易懂、跃然纸上的漫画。而且，听妈妈讲故事的形式，还会使小朋友在感受中医药文化的书香画韵之外，品味到母子生活的欢愉和阅读的乐趣。

本书分为果实类、全草类、花类、根茎类、种子类 5 章，共计 40 余个小故事。采用中英文对照的形式，让不同人群更好地感受中草药的魅力，充满了趣味性和科学性，让家长在陪孩子阅读时，可以更多地了解中草药。英文部分可以增加本书的实用性，让这本书能够跨越地域的界限、跨越语言的障碍，将中医药文化传播到世界各地。

本书由上海市浦东新区光明中医医院牵头编写，获得了 2016 年度"浦东新区中医药研发创新专项"项目（编号：PDZYYFCX -201603）立项资助，得到了上海中医药大学、浦东新区卫生和计划生育委员会中医药发展与科教处、浦东新区中医药发展中心、浦东新区中医药创新促进中心等单位的大力协助。本书虽然经过多次修订，但内容可能还有不少疏漏，真诚希望各位读者斧正。

编　者

2018 年 4 月

目录 Contents

果实类
Fruits

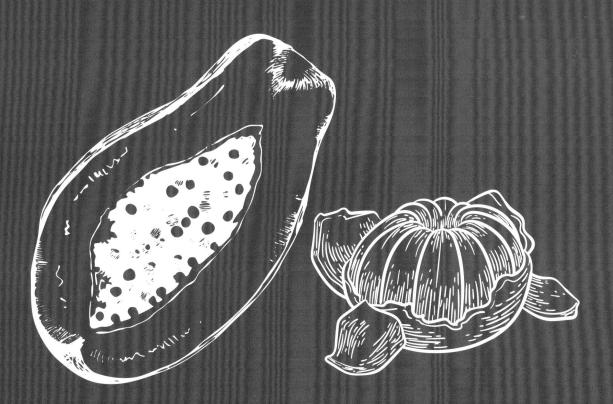

佛手

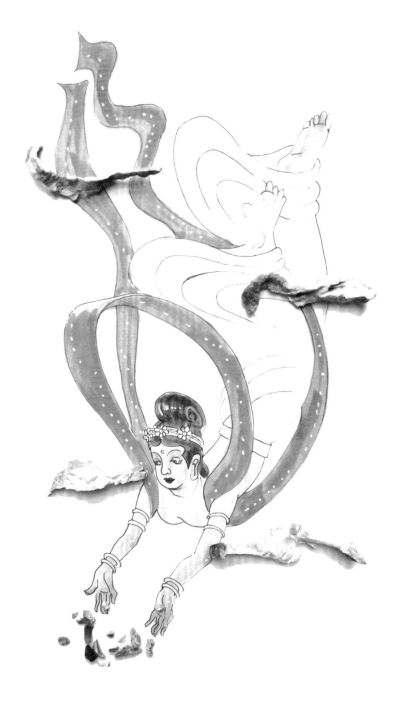

很久很久以前，在金华山下住着狐狸一家，狐狸爸爸经常出差，狐狸妈妈每天辛苦地做着家务，照顾着狐狸宝宝。

有一天，狐狸妈妈做完家务，累坏了，感觉胸口闷闷的，肚子胀胀的。狐狸宝宝看妈妈病了，心里很着急。这天夜里，狐狸宝宝梦见了仙女，仙女给了他像美丽的小手一般的果子，并对狐狸宝宝说："金华山上有这样的金果，能治好你妈妈的病。"

第二天，狐狸宝宝鼓起勇气爬到了金华山上。山顶开满了金色的小花，树上长满了金灿灿的橘子，漫山遍野清香扑鼻，狐狸宝宝走近一看，树上的橘子正是梦里仙女给他的金果。狐狸宝宝摘下了金果带回家，狐狸妈妈吃了金果，觉得胸口很舒服，肚子也不胀了。

狐狸宝宝和狐狸妈妈都很高兴，就把金果的种子种在了院子里。种子慢慢长成果树。秋天到了，果树结了好多果子，香气吸引了邻居们，狐狸宝宝和狐狸妈妈就把树上的果子摘下来和邻居一起分享。

邻居们听了狐狸宝宝的故事，认为他梦里的那位仙女就是观世音菩萨，这金灿灿的果子就像她美丽的手，所以大家都叫这果子"佛手"。

Fo Shou

Once upon a time, a fox family lived in Jin Hua Mountain. The fox father often went on business trips, leaving the mother doing the housework and taking care of the baby alone.

One day, after finishing the housework, the mother fox felt exhausted, with chest tightness and abdominal distension. The baby fox was very worried. That night, the baby fox dreamt of a fairy giving him a beautiful small fruit that shaped like a hand. The fairy told the baby fox: "This golden fruit can cure your mother's disease. It grows in Jin Hua Mountain." The next day, the baby fox summoned up courage and climbed up to Jin Hua Mountain. Full of golden flowers and trees hanging with golden fruits, the mountain top was filled with fragrances. The baby fox went closer and surprisingly found that the fruits on the trees were the exact the golden fruit that the fairy gave him in the dream. The baby fox picked the golden fruits and brought them home to his mother. After taking them, her chest discomfort and her abdominal distension was gone.

The baby fox and the mother fox were delighted, and planted the seeds in the yard. When the seeds grew into fruit trees, their aroma attracted the neighbors. By the fall, the baby fox and the mother fox shared the fruits with the neighbors.

After the neighbors heard the whole story, they all thought the fairy he dreamt of was warm-hearted Bodhisattva and the golden fruit was like her beautiful hand. Therefore, everybody called this fruit "Fo Shou"(literally means Bodhisattva's hand).

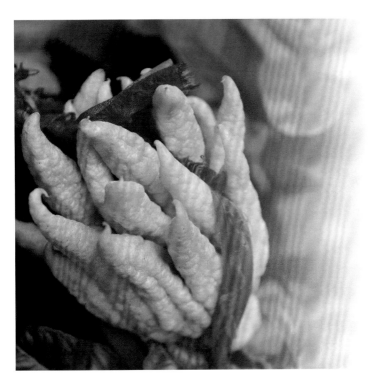

佛手 果实类

用药部位	果实
开花时间	4～5月
生长环境	温暖湿润、阳光充足的热带地区
味道	辣、苦、甜

连翘

相传，五千年前有个叫岐伯的老爷爷喜欢种药、采药。他有个孙女名叫连翘。

一天，岐伯和孙女连翘在山上采药时，发现了一种从没见过的果子，看起来很好吃的样子，于是岐伯就摘下来尝了一口。没想到这果子有毒，岐伯倒在了地上，虚弱地喊着："连翘救命！连翘救命！"连翘发现爷爷中毒严重，有生命危险，泪流满面地抱着爷爷哭喊。好久都没人过来，无奈之下，连翘急中生智摘了一把身边的绿叶，在手里揉碎后塞进爷爷的嘴里。过了一会儿，爷爷慢慢苏醒过来，再一会儿，爷爷竟然可以站起来了。

后来，岐伯用孙女的名字命名这种植物，把它叫作"连翘"，这个故事也因此流传至今。

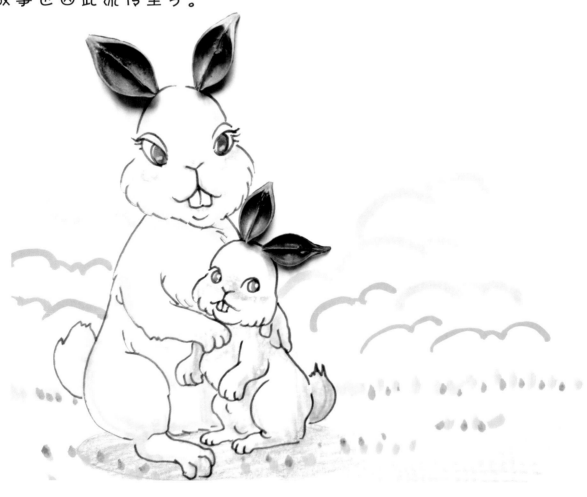

Lian Qiao

It was said that five thousand years ago, an old man named Qi Bo liked to plant herbs and collect herbs. He had a granddaughter called Lian Qiao.

One day, when he and his granddaughter were picking herbs on the mountain, they found a fruit that they had never seen before. He thought that it may be delicious, so he picked one and took a bite, but the fruit was poisonous. Qi Bo fell down and nearly became unconscious. He kept calling his granddaughter in a low voice. Knowing that grandpa was poisoned and at risks, Lian Qiao embraced grandpa and cried for help. However, after crying for a long time, no one came. She was so anxious that she grabbed a handful of leaves beside her, grinded them in the hand and stuffed them into grandfather's mouth. After a while, Qi Bo slowly became conscious. A moment after swallowing the green leaves, he stood up.

Qi Bo named this green leaves after his granddaughter Lian Qiao. Therefore, the story also passed down.

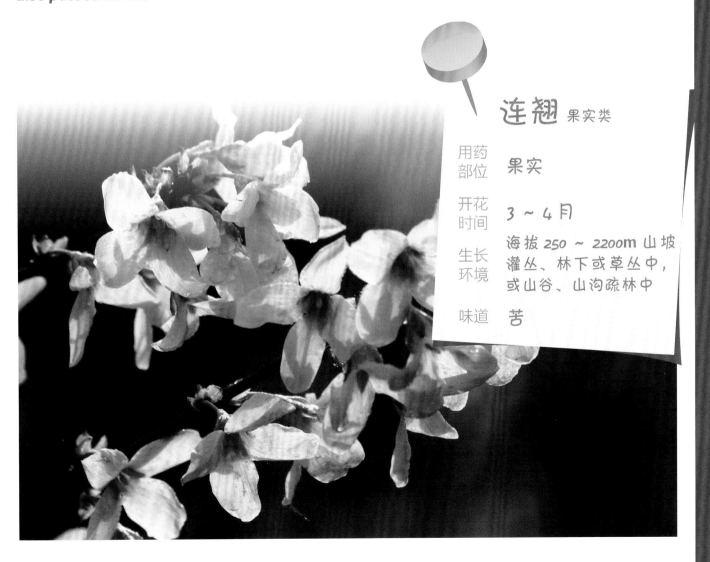

连翘 果实类

用药部位 果实

开花时间 3 ~ 4月

生长环境 海拔 250 ~ 2200m 山坡灌丛、林下或草丛中，或山谷、山沟疏林中

味道 苦

陈皮

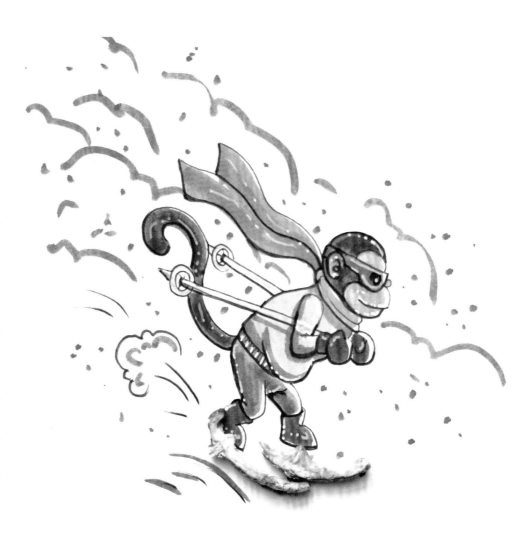

一天，名医华佗乘船去江西行医。突然，一阵阵大风吹过来，华佗觉得自己开始发热，不停地咳嗽，嘴巴也很干，可是他身上已经没有药了。

正在这时候，船经过一个岸边，岸上的橘子树上结满了好吃的橘子。华佗想，药丸没了，摘点橘子吃吃，至少也能解渴，回到船上，他连皮带肉一连吃了好几个。到了晚上，华佗突然觉得咳嗽好多了。他有点奇怪，自己没吃药，咳嗽怎么好些了呢？难道橘子能治咳嗽？第二天，船上的两名船夫也染上了感冒，咳嗽起来，华佗便拿出橘子给他们吃。

谁知道，两名船夫吃后，一个咳嗽好了，另一个仍咳个不停。华佗很纳闷，仔细追问才得知原来不再咳嗽的一位船夫是将橘子连皮带肉一起吃，而无效的一人是只吃橘肉没吃橘皮。华佗突然想道：难道橘皮可以止咳？之后，华佗每次吃橘子时，都把橘皮留下。

几个月后，华佗行医归来，发现那些橘皮都被风吹干了。一天，正好有人感冒咳嗽前来就诊，华佗便把干的橘皮煎水让病人服用，没想到效果更棒。就这样，陈皮成了一种重要的用来止咳的中药材。

Chen Pi

One day, the famous physician Hua Tuo went to Jiang Xi to visit patients by boat. Suddenly, a burst of wind blew. Hua Tuo began to have a fever with cough and dry mouth. However, he didn't bring any medicines along with him.

At this time, he noticed that there were delicious tangerines growing on tangerine trees on the shore. Hua Tuo thought that since there were no pills, he could still pick some tangerines to quench thirst. He returned to the boat with some tangerines and took several even with the peels. At night, he noticed that he was coughing less. He was surprised that he could stop coughing without medicines. Was it the tangerine that can stop coughing? The next day, the two crew men also caught a cold and coughed, and Hua Tuo took out tangerines for them.

After eating tangerines, one stopped coughing and the other didn't. Hua Tuo was confused. It turned out that one only took the tangerine fruits, while another took the whole tangerine along with the peels. Hua Tuo suddenly realized that maybe tangerine peels can stop cough. After wards, every time Hua Tuo had tangerines, he would save the tangerine peels.

A few months later, he returned home and found that the tangerines peels had been air-dried. One day, someone suffering a cold and cough visited him, Hua Tuo boiled the dried tangerine peels and asked the patient to take it. Surprisingly, the therapeutic effects were even better. In this way, Hua Tuo discovered the tangerine peel as a medicine. From then on, tangerine peel (Chen Pi) has become an important herb in Chinese Medicine.

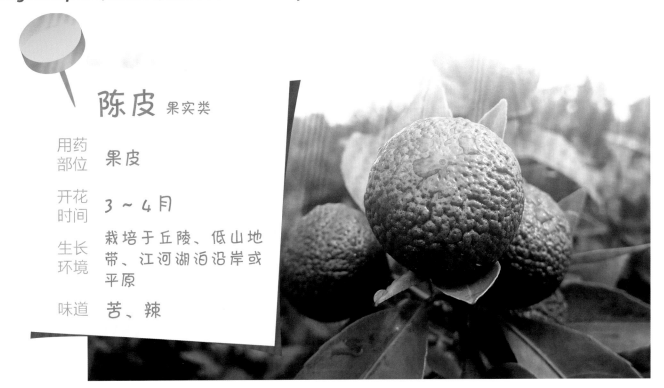

陈皮 果实类

用药部位	果皮
开花时间	3～4月
生长环境	栽培于丘陵、低山地带、江河湖泊沿岸或平原
味道	苦、辣

枳壳

　　有个读中学的小胖子，因为喜欢吃东西，所以越来越胖。小胖子每天不停地吃着各种东西：蛋糕、巧克力、炸猪排……时间长了，小胖子觉得自己时常会胸闷、腹胀。

　　有一天，老师带同学们到淮北秋游。大家来到一片果园，一起玩摘橘子的游戏。一位农民伯伯看到小胖子摘橘子很吃力，看起来身体有些不舒服，问明情况后便对他说："这里的果子可不是橘子，橘子是长在淮河南边的，长在北边就叫做枳子。你拿回去晒干它，用它的壳煮水喝，可以治好你的病。"

　　小胖子拿了农民伯伯给的枳子回家，让妈妈帮忙晒干了枳子，用它的壳儿煮水喝了几天。小胖子放了好多大臭屁，胸口舒服了很多，胃里也不胀了，感觉轻松多了。小胖子暗暗下决心一定要减肥，向农民伯伯学习，多种一些像枳子一样可以作为中药材的水果，帮助和自己有一样症状的小胖子们。

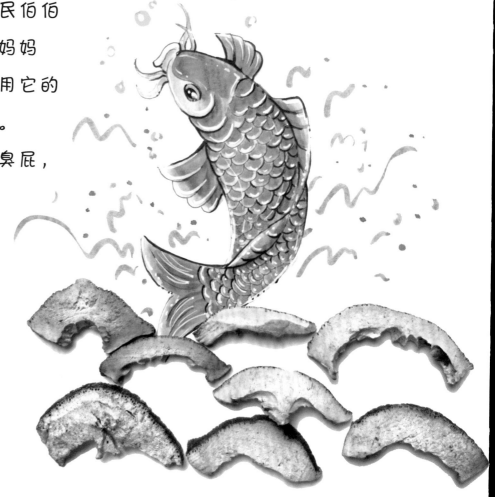

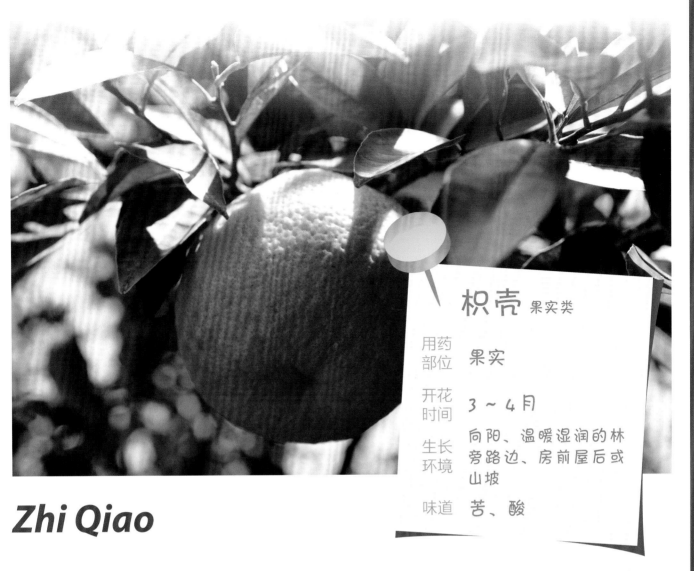

枳壳 果实类

用药部位	果实
开花时间	3～4月
生长环境	向阳、温暖湿润的林旁路边、房前屋后或山坡
味道	苦、酸

Zhi Qiao

There was a little fat boy who was in middle school. He liked eating, so he became fatter and fatter. Every day he ate all sorts of things, such as cakes, chocolates and fried pork chops. In the long term, the little boy always had chest tightness and stomach distension.

One day, the teacher led the class to Huai Bei for an autumn tour. Everyone came to an orchard picked tangerines. A farmer saw the little fat boy pick tangerines with difficulty and the boy looked uncomfortable. Then the farmer told the boy: "The fruit here is not a tangerine. Tangerine grows in the south of Huai He River. The one grows in the north is called trifoliate orange. You can take it back, dry it and boil it with its shell, and it will cure your problem."

He took the trifoliate oranges home, the fat boy asked his mother to dry them and boil them in water. A few days later, after passing gas, the boy felt much better as if the big stone situating in the chest was gone and the stomach distension was relieved. The boy secretly made a resolution to lose weight and to learn from the farmer by planting more trifoliate oranges which can act as herbs to help over weight boys like himself.

山楂

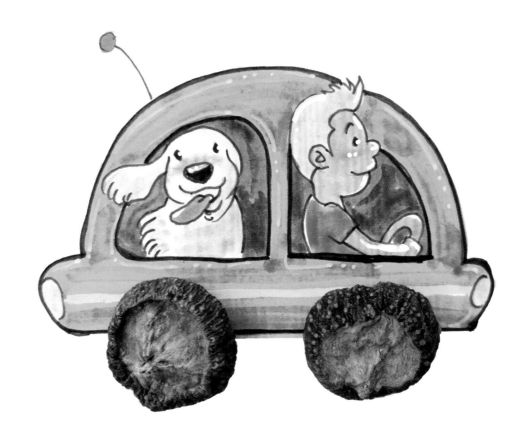

　　唐代天宝年间，唐玄宗的宠妃杨玉环患了腹胀病，出现脘腹胀满、不思饮食、大便泄泻等症状。经过很多太医诊治，用遍了名贵药材也不见好转，唐玄宗非常着急，只得张榜招名医。一天，有位道士路过皇宫，当即揭榜为皇妃治病。道士检查了贵妃的脉象和舌苔，开了处方后扬长而去。皇帝对此将信将疑，但还是照方遣药。谁知用药不到半月，皇妃的病果真好了。据说，方中主要药物是山楂。原来，杨贵妃为使肌肤细嫩光滑，经常食用一道叫作"阿胶羹"的药膳。因阿胶药性滋补，一直服用可导致腹胀，妨碍消化。经道士诊治后，她终于明白了自己的病根，此后服食阿胶羹的同时，常佐食些山楂，果然旧病不发，体安神爽。

Shan Zha

In Tiao Bao period (742—756) of tang dynasty, Yang Yuhuan, the most favored concubine of Emperor Tang Xuanzong suffered from abdominal distension, with symptoms of abdominal distension, no appetite for food and drinks, and diarrhea. After seeing many imperial physicians and taking many rare medicines, Yang didn't feel better. Emperor Tang Xuanzong was very anxious, so he posted an imperial notice to find famous and excellent physicians. One day, a Taoist priest passed by the imperial palace and took off the notice and entered the palace. After taking the pulse and observing the tongue of Yang, the Taoist priest prescribed a formula and went away. The emperor was skeptical, but he collected the medicines as prescribed. Surprisingly, after less than half a month, Yang got recovered. The main herb of the formula was hawthorn. It was said that in order to win the favor of the emperor, Yang always took a herb called E Jiao Porridge (E Jiao: donkey gelatin) for smoother and tender skin. As E Jiao is tonic, long-term intake will lead to abdominal distension and indigestion. Therefore, after the priest's diagnosis and treatment, Yang knew her problem. Since then, when she was served E Jiao porridge, she would took some hawthorn at the same time. Indeed, the disease never occurred to her again and she felt more comfortable.

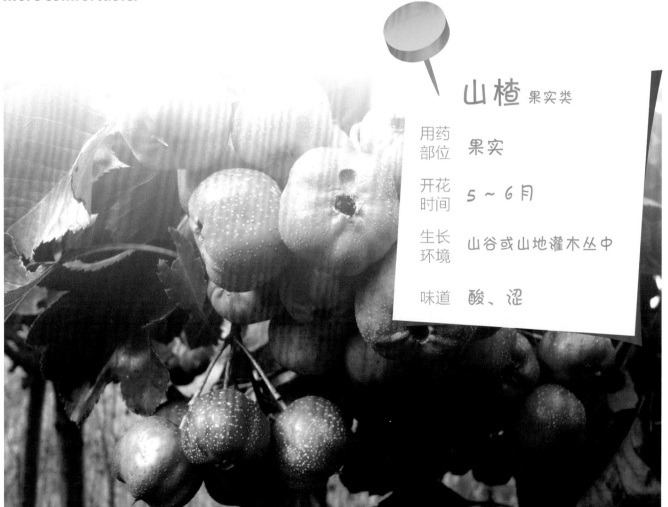

山楂 果实类

用药
部位　果实

开花
时间　5 ～ 6 月

生长
环境　山谷或山地灌木丛中

味道　酸、涩

木瓜

　　宋代名医许叔微在《普济本事方》中记载了一则有趣的故事：安徽有个叫顾安中的人外出，突发腿脚肿痛，不能行走，只好乘船回家。在船上，他将两脚放在一包装货的袋子上休息，下船时突然发现自己腿脚肿胀疼痛的症状竟然缓解了许多，感到十分惊奇，就问船家袋中装的是什么，船家回答说袋子里装的是木瓜。顾安中回家后，买了一些木瓜切片，装于袋中，每日将脚放在上面，不久，他的腿脚病居然痊愈了。原来，木瓜有治疗风湿痹痛的神奇功效。

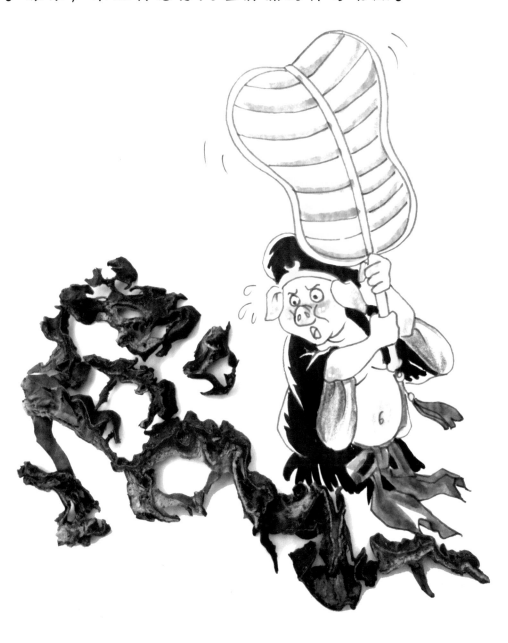

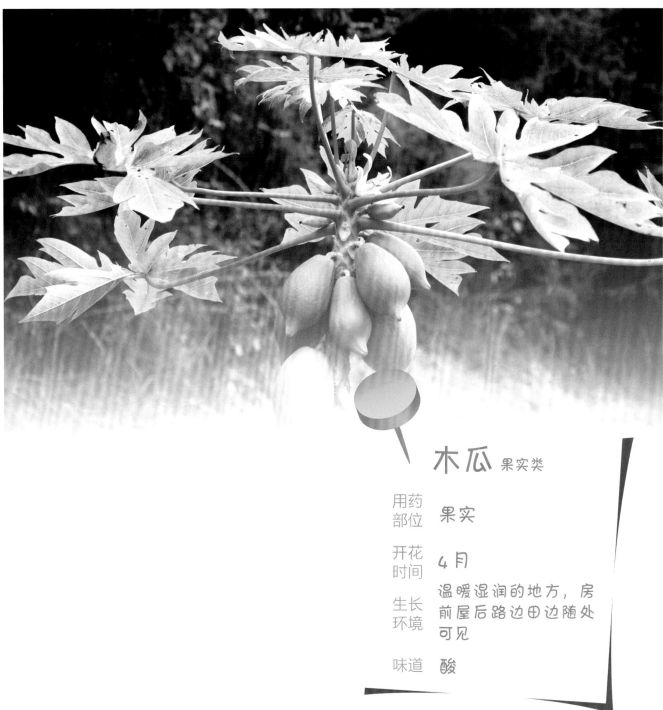

木瓜 果实类

用药部位　果实

开花时间　4月

生长环境　温暖湿润的地方，房前屋后路边田边随处可见

味道　酸

Mu Gua

Xu Shuwei, a famous physician in song dynasty, recorded an interesting story in his book Ben Shi Fang. Here is the story: In An Hui province, a man named Gu An Zhong suddenly had a swollen and painful leg and could not walk home. So he had to take a boat home. On the boat, he put both feet on a pack of goods. When he got off the boat, he found the leg was much better. With surprise, he went to ask what was in the bag. The crew answered it was papaya in the bag. After he returned home, Gu bought some papayas, sliced them and put them in a bag. Then he put his feet on the bag every day. Soon, he was cured. In fact papaya has the magical effects in treating rheumatoid pains.

桑椹

　　相传楚汉相争时，刘邦曾在徐州被项羽打得一败涂地，好不容易冲出重围，率领骑兵逃跑。没想到前有高山挡路，后有追兵堵截，走投无路之下，刘邦一行人匆忙躲进一个阴暗的山洞里。项羽追到洞前，见洞口都是蜘蛛网，觉得一定不会有人闯入，转身向别处追去。

　　刘邦虽然躲过一劫，但因为受到惊吓，头痛、头晕的老毛病复发了。他觉得天旋地转，腰酸腿软，甚至大便也拉不出来了，很痛苦。一天，刘邦行军经过桑树林，发现树上结了很多桑椹。为了填饱肚子，刘邦只能摘下桑椹充饥。奇怪的是，连着吃了几日桑椹，他的头痛、头晕的症状竟不知不觉地消失了，大便也能够顺利排出来了，整个人都精神清爽，身体强劲有力。

　　后来刘邦成了汉朝的开国皇帝，仍不忘桑椹的救命之恩。御医顺着他的心意，将桑椹加蜂蜜熬成膏，让他常年养生服用来保持身体健康。

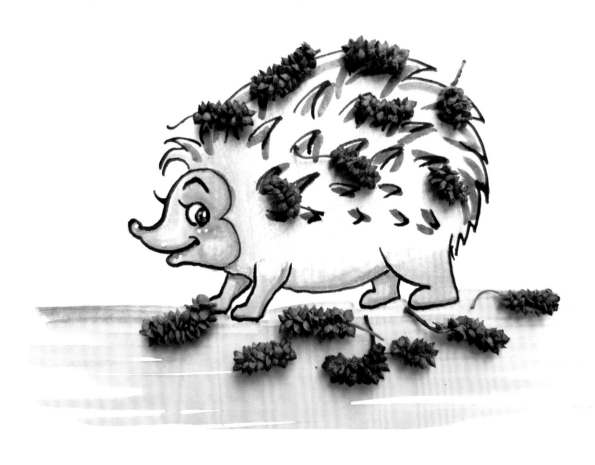

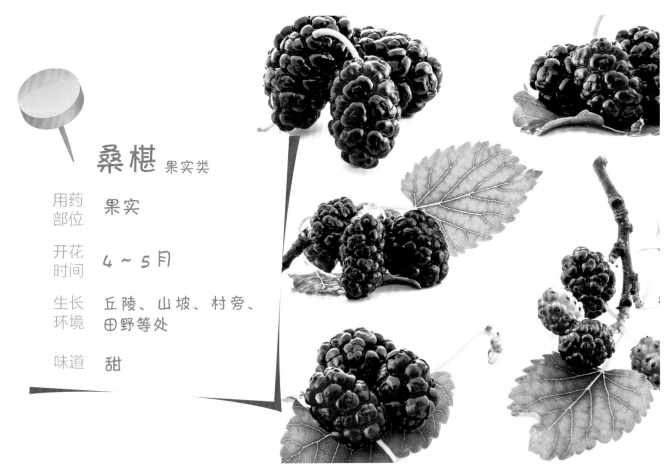

桑椹 果实类

用药部位	果实
开花时间	4 ~ 5月
生长环境	丘陵、山坡、村旁、田野等处
味道	甜

Sang Shen

Legend has it that in the war between Chu and Han Dynasties, Liu Bang was terribly beaten in Xu Zhou by Xiang Yu. After getting through the close siege, Liu Bang fled with his cavalries. Unexpectedly, he was trapped with high mountains before him and enemies behind. In desperation, Liu Bang and his cavalries hurried to hide in a dark cave. When Xiang Yu got to the cave, he saw that the hole was covered with cobwebs, so he thought no one broke in. Then he left.

Although escaped the hunting, Liu Bang suffered from the recurrence of headache and dizziness because of shock. He felt the world was whirling. Moreover he was tortured by sore lumbar, weak legs and constipation. On the way to escape, they passed a forest of mulberry trees. There were many mulberry fruits. In order to fill his stomach, Liu Bang had to take the mulberry fruits. Oddly, he took them successively for a few days, the headache and dizziness got recovered. And the constipation was also relieved. He felt more relaxed and more energetic.

Later, after Liu Bang became the founding emperor of Han Dynasty, he still remembered the help of mulberry. The imperial physician knew that, so he made a paste with mulberr fruits and honey, and sent it to Liu Bang for health maintenance.

白豆蔻

古时候有一个郎中结婚多年一直没有孩子，老年时才喜得一女，却不想女儿总是吐乳、腹泻。郎中辨证是脾虚胃寒，他试着给女儿熬了几副中药，可女儿根本喝不下去。有一次他想硬灌几口下去，结果惹得女儿频频呕吐。从此他再也不敢逼女儿喝中药了。

一天，郎中在清理中草药时，女儿爬了过来，抓着颗白豆蔻把玩。白豆蔻果实饱满，非常好看。一开始郎中也没管她，可后来女儿竟然把白豆蔻往嘴里塞，郎中怎么都拦不住。郎中突发奇想，决定就单用白豆蔻煎汤试试。万万没想到，这单方用对了，女儿竟然肯喝一些白豆蔻汤。更令郎中惊喜的是，孩子喝了这汤之后喝奶也积极多了，慢慢地身体也好了起来。

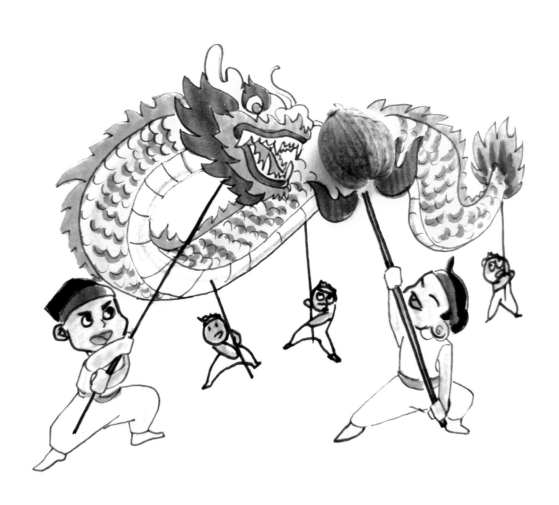

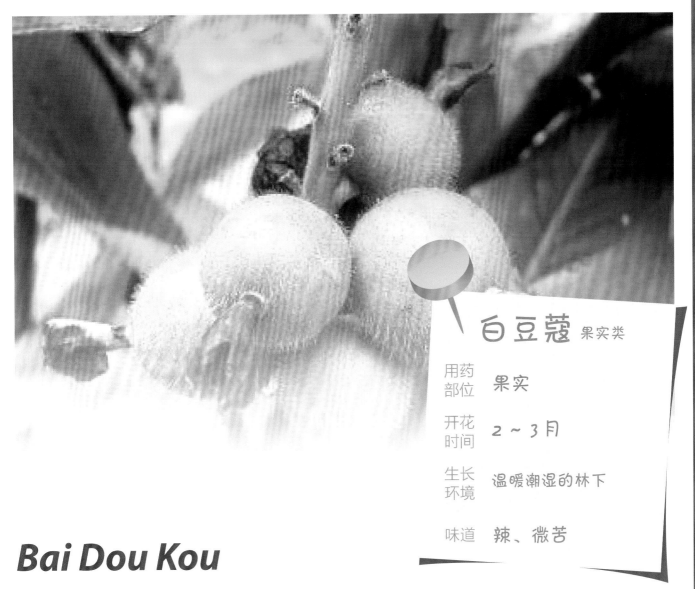

白豆蔻 果实类

用药部位	果实
开花时间	2 ~ 3月
生长环境	温暖潮湿的林下
味道	辣、微苦

Bai Dou Kou

In ancient times, there was a young physician who had never had any children after marriage. When he was old, he finally had a daughter. However, the little girl always spit out milk and suffered from diarrhea. After pattern identification, it was spleen deficiency and stomach coldness. yet. The girl did not like to take the decoction. He tried to boil some decoction for her, but the girl couldn't swallow it. Sometimes, he opened her mouth and tried to pour the decoction in it, but the girl vomited for a long time. Since then, he didn't dare to force her to take Chinese medicine.

One day, while the physician was cleaning the Chinese herbs, the daughter climbed over and played with some Bai Dou Kou. It is no wonder that the girl liked to play with Bai Dou Kou for it is round and good-looking. Therefore, at the beginning, the physician didn't stop her. Nevertheless, the girl even stuffed herself with Bai Dou Kou. The physician hurriedly stopped her. But the kid didn't care and she stuffed everything she saw into her mouth. He suddenly came up with an idea that he can boil Bai Dou Kou for his daughter. If she still didn't drink it, he would give up. Surprisingly, the therapy worked and she drank some. After taking the decoction, the little girl started to drink milk and began to get better.

枸杞子

　　相传很久以前，卫宁这个地方是一片汪洋大海。大禹用开山大斧劈开青铜古山来填补大海，卫宁大地就慢慢出现了，这里土肥水美、阳光充足、四季分明、五谷丰登。

　　失去海洋的北海龙王很生气，将大禹告上天庭，说大禹侵犯他的领地，北海越来越干旱，龙子龙孙没地方可以居住。玉皇大帝不知人间这样巨大的变化，派王母娘娘和太上老君下界用"五色土"堵住了山口，想让卫宁平原再变成汪洋。

　　善良的王母娘娘下界看到这里的百姓安居乐业，不忍心让这里再变成大海，于是将"五色土"抛在了山的南边。为了继续造福凡间百姓，她把自己的红耳坠留在了人间，神奇的红耳坠变成很多红灿灿的小果实，当地人们吃了这些小果实后，干活更有力气，不会腰酸，眼睛也变得更加明亮，这就是造福人类的"红宝"枸杞子，它的别名就叫"红耳坠"。

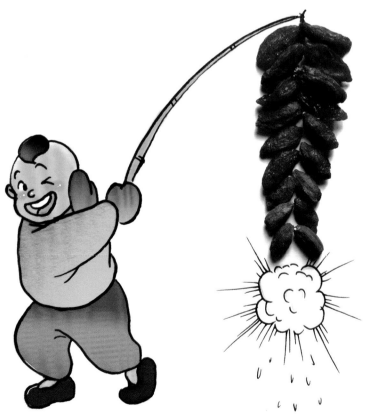

Gou Qi Zi

Long long ago, Wei Ning was a vast ocean. Da Yu waved a big axes to chop the ancient bronze mountain to fill up the sea. Gradually, the land of Wei Ning emerged, with fertile soil, rich water, abundant sunlight, distinct four seasons and a good harvest.

The king of north sea was furious for losing the ocean, so he accused Da Yu of invading his territory and filled the ocean with mountain rocks. As a result, the north sea became drier and drier, and his generation had no place to live. The Jade Emperor did not know the great change of the world, so he sent the Queen of Heaven and the Supreme Lord to block the mountain gate with "five color earth", trying to change the plain of Wei Ning back into an ocean.

When they got to the earth, the kind Queen of Heaven saw the people here live in peace and harmony and she couldn't bear to let this turn into ocean again. Therefore, she threw the "five color earth" on the south side of the mountain. In order to keep bringing benefits to the people, she left her red eardrop on the earth. Magically, bright red fruits began to grow on the red eardrop. The local people who took them became more strengthful. Besides, their waist soreness was gone and eyes were brighter. These fruits were Chinese wolfberry fruits that do goods to people. We also call them red eardrops.

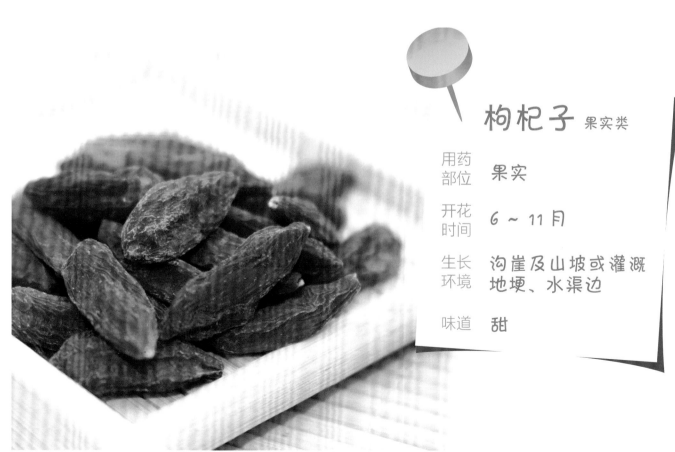

枸杞子 果实类

用药部位	果实
开花时间	6 ~ 11 月
生长环境	沟崖及山坡或灌溉地埂、水渠边
味道	甜

女贞子

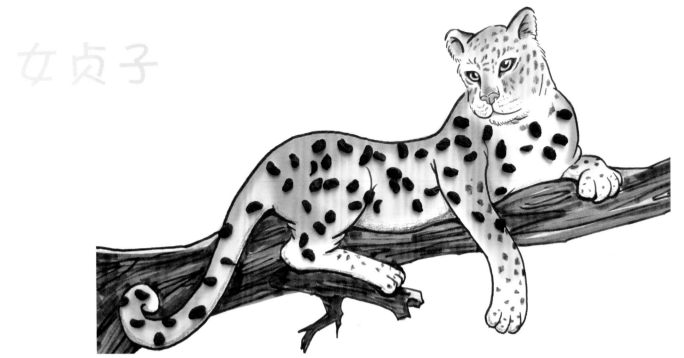

从前有个善良的姑娘叫贞子，嫁给了一个老实的农夫，两人十分恩爱。那时候经常打仗，贞子的丈夫也被抓去当兵，一走就没了音信。贞子一个人万分凄凉，一天，同村有个当兵的捎信回来说贞子的丈夫已经战死。贞子听后，当时就昏死过去，她一连十几天不吃不喝，只是哭。一天，贞子睁开眼睛拉着隔壁二姐的手说道："好姐姐，我死后，你就在我坟前栽一棵冬青树。万一他回来找我，这棵树能表明我的心意！"不久，贞子就病死了。

二姐在贞子的坟前栽了一棵冬青。几年过去了，一天，贞子的丈夫突然回了家。听说了贞子的事情，丈夫十分伤心，一头扑在坟上，哭了三天三夜，泪水洒湿了冬青树。丈夫因为伤心过度，从此生了病。说来奇怪，贞子坟前的冬青树被泪水淋过后，忽然开花了，还结出了许多豆粒大的果子。因为平常的冬青树从不开花结果，人们就都说贞子死后成仙了，她坟上的树也成了仙树。这事被贞子的丈夫知道了，他来到坟前看到满树的小果子，心里一动：莫非这棵树真得了妻子的仙气不成？那么，吃了这果子不是也能成仙吗？这样就能和贞子见面了。想到这里，他摘下果子就吃。可吃了几天也没成仙，更没见到贞子。不过，他的病却慢慢好了。

于是，人们知道贞子坟前的树上结的果子是药，为了纪念贞子就给它取了一个名字，叫"女贞子"。

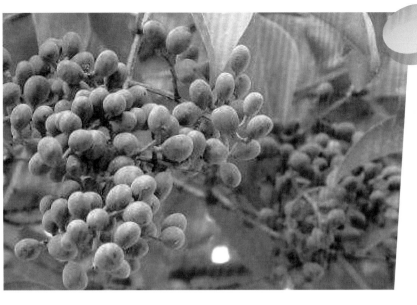

女贞子 果实类

用药部位	果实
开花时间	6 ~ 7 月
生长环境	海拔 2900m 下的疏林或密林中
味道	甜中微辣

Nv Zhen Zi

Once upon a time, there was a kind girl named Zhen Zi. She married to an honest farmer and they lived a happy life together. In those war-ridden years, many men, including her husband, were captured as soldiers. After his absence, she had never heard a word about him. She lived a miserable life alone. One day, the soldier from the same village sent a message back saying that her husband had passed away. On hearing this, Zhen Zi passed out immediately. She did nothing but crying continuously for more than ten days. One day, she opened her eyes and said to the elder woman next door: "Dear sister, if I die, you may plant a Holly tree in front of my grave. In case he comes back, this tree will show my heart!" Later, Zhen Zi died.

The elder sister planted a Holly tree in front of her grave. A few years passed. One day, her husband came home suddenly. When he approached the Holly tree, he threw himself on the grave and cried for three days and three nights. The tears wet the whole tree. Due to great grief, the husband became ill. Strangely, the holly tree in front of the grave suddenly blossomed and even bore soybean-shaped fruits after the husband shed tears on it. The villagers were confused, for the holly never blossoms. Therefore, rumors came that Zhen Zi became the immortal after she died, and the tree before her grave became a immortal tree. Hearing this rumor, the husband came to the grave and did see the little fruits hanging on the tree. He thought: "Does this tree really get the immortal power from my wife? If so, can I become an immortal after taking these fruits? If this is true, I can meet her again." Thinking of this, he picked the fruits and took them. After taking them for several days, he didn't become an immortal, nor did he see his wife. But he was slowly getting better.

So people knew that the tree in front of the grave was a herbal tree. Since then, gave it the name of "Nv Zhen Zi".

金樱子

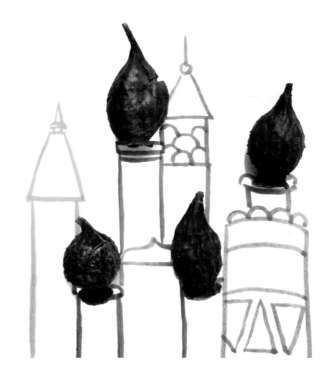

　　从前有一个安静的小镇，镇上住着小男孩贝贝一家，贝贝已经十岁了，可是他仍然很容易尿床。看到贝贝家晒着的床单，小伙伴们就知道贝贝又尿床了，所以都叫他"尿床大王"。

　　贝贝妈妈觉得贝贝一定是做噩梦了，才容易尿床，所以在贝贝睡前给他讲故事逗他开心，可是贝贝还是会尿床。妈妈又觉得贝贝可能是吃得不好，营养不够才会尿床，于是每天都给贝贝吃各种好吃又有营养的饭菜，可是都没有用。

　　有一天，镇上来了一位带着宝葫芦的老中医，贝贝妈妈赶紧去向老中医寻求帮助，老中医从自己的葫芦里找出一种像金色樱桃般的小果子，让贝贝妈妈给贝贝煮水喝。连续喝了几天，贝贝渐渐地不尿床了，妈妈也不用再那么辛苦地洗床单了。

　　小伙伴们都觉得很好奇，"尿床大王"怎么不尿床了呢？于是他们就去找到那位正要告别小镇的老中医问："是什么灵丹妙药治好了贝贝的尿床呀？"老中医笑着从宝葫芦里掏出那种金色小樱桃般的果子，给大家看："治好贝贝尿床病的，就是这种中药，你们看像不像金色的樱桃，我们就叫他'金樱子'吧！"

Jin Ying Zi

Once upon a time there was a quiet and serene town where a little boy named Bei Bei lived with his family. At the age of 10, Bei Bei was still easy to wet his bed. When the neighbors saw the bed sheets, they knew that Bei Bei was bed-wetting, so everyone called him "bed-wetting king".

Considering that bed-wetting was due to the nightmare, Bei Bei's mother told him bedtime stories to make him happy. However, it didn't work. Thinking that it may be caused by poor nutrition, his mother provided him all kinds of delicious and nutritious food every day, but it was also useless.

One day, an old physician of traditional Chinese medicine with a gourd came to the town. Bei Bei's mother hurried to seek help from him. The old physician took a golden cherry-like fruit from his gourd and told Bei Bei's mother to boil it. After Bei Bei drank the soup boiled with the fruits for a few days, Bei Bei gradually stopped bed-wetting, and her mother did not have to wash the sheets so hard.

The friends were all curious about why the bed-wetting king didn't wet the bed? So they asked the old physician who was about to leave the town: "what magic elixir cured Bei Bei's bed-wetting?" The old physician smiled and presented the golden cherry-like fruit, saying that: "It was the Chinese herb that cured Bei Bei's bed-wetting. Look, it looks like a golden cherry. So it is called Jin Ying Zi (Jin literally means golden; Ying refers to cherry)."

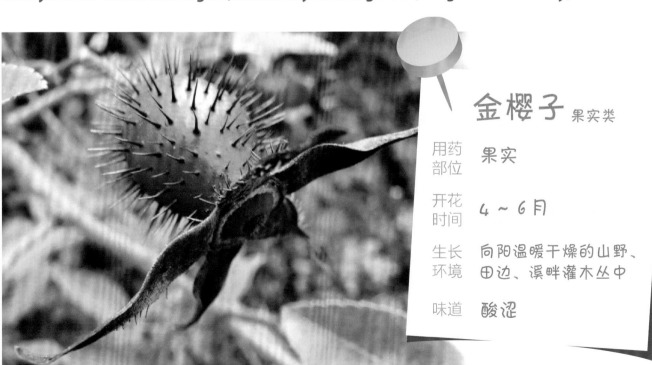

金樱子 果实类

用药部位　果实

开花时间　4～6月

生长环境　向阳温暖干燥的山野、田边、溪畔灌木丛中

味道　酸涩

益智仁

相传很久以前，有一个富豪，到五十岁才有了一个儿子，取名叫来福。来福这孩子跟别的小孩不一样，自小体弱多病，性格木讷，常常尿床。为了给儿子看病，富豪把附近的有名的医生都请去家里，结果什么原因都查不出，病情自然也没有好转。

有一天，一个老道士经过这个地方，听说了来福治病的事情，他找到富豪拿起手里的拐杖往南边一指，说："离这里八千里的地方有一种果树，上面结的果实可以治好孩子的病。"说完还在地上画了一幅画，画中是一棵大树，叶子狭长舒展，树的顶部长着椭圆形的果实。富豪请了很多人去外面寻找，功夫不负有心人，果实终于被寻回来了。来福吃到采摘回来的果实后，很少尿床，而且变得开朗活泼、聪颖可爱，后来还上了学堂。在十八岁那年参加了科举考试中了状元。

来福的故事在当地传开了，老百姓把治愈他疾病的果实取名为"状元果"，同时也由于它能使人头脑聪明，所以也叫它"益智仁"。

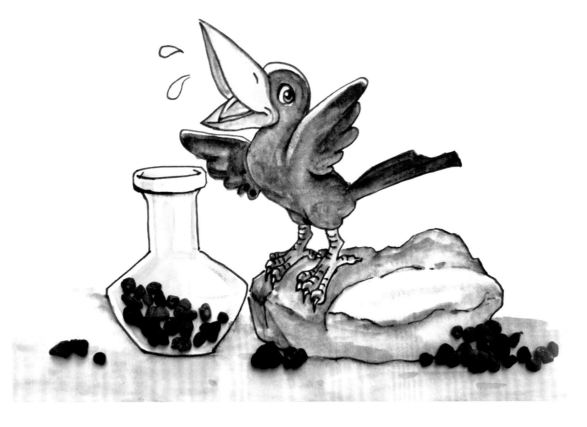

Yi Zhi Ren

Once upon a time, there was a rich man who finally had a son when he was at the age of fifty. He named the boy Lai Fu (literally means good fortune for the boy). However, unlike other children, the boy was weak and sick. He looked dull and wet bed sometime. He often forgot the previous number when counting to the next one. In order to treat his son, the rich man had invited all the famous physicians nearby. However, they couldn't find out what was wrong, and the treatment didn't work.

One day, a Taoist priest heard this when passing by. After inquiring something about the boy, the priest pointed his stick to the south and said: "There's a kindof tree eight thousand miles away,and its fruit can cure the boy's disease." Then he drew the tree on the ground. The long and narrow leaves grew extended. At the top of the tree, oval fruits were grown. The rich man sent a lot of people to find it. Hard work pays off. After the boy took the fruits, he seldom wets his bed again, more cheerful and cleverer. Later, he went to school and took the imperial examination at the age of eighteen.

The locals all knew about his cleverness, and they named the fruits curing him "the very best fruits". As it can make people clever, it is also called it "Yi Zhi Ren" (literally means the kernels making you clever).

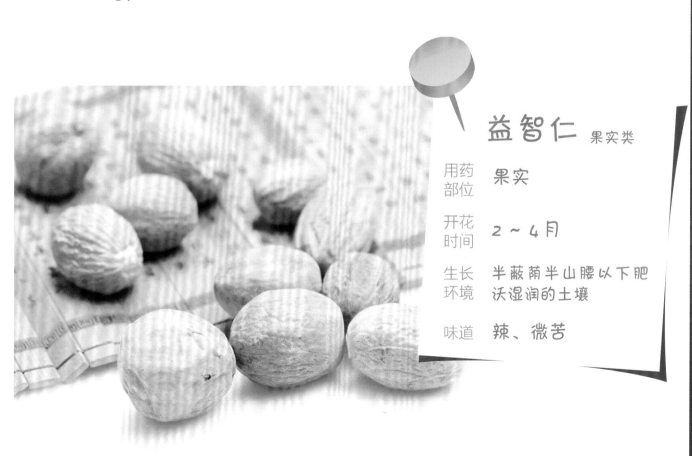

益智仁 果实类

用药部位　果实

开花时间　2～4月

生长环境　半蔽荫半山腰以下肥沃湿润的土壤

味道　辣、微苦

全草类

Herbs

夏枯草

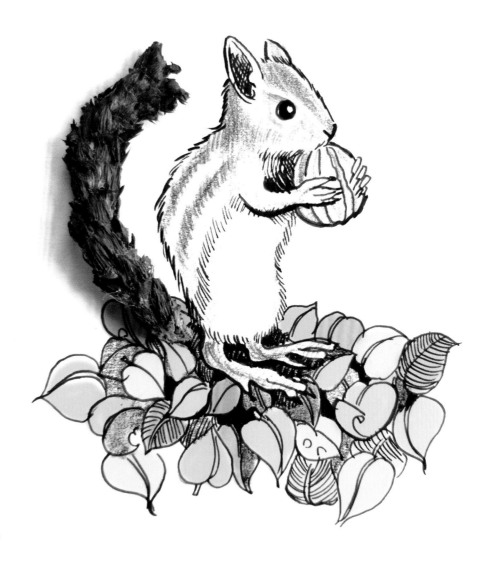

有个小伙子叫小明，非常勤劳，而且热心助人。小明和村里的小花感情很好，但是小花家人不同意小花嫁给小明，因为小明脖子粗大，就像青蛙一样难看。小明看了很多的医生，吃了很多中药都没有好，因此很苦恼。

有一天，一位衣服破旧，面黄肌瘦的老人倒在了小明家的门口，小明看到后，不仅没有嫌弃还把老人背回了家。过了一段时间，老人身体慢慢好了，他见到小明不开心，就问小明："小明，你怎么不开心啊？"

小明回答道："爷爷，因为我脖子很粗，样子难看，我心爱女孩儿的家人不同意把她嫁给我。医生也治不好我的病，因此很着急。"

老人知道小明是个好小伙。于是，告诉小明："山上有一种草，紫颜色的，看上去像小虫子，这种草对你的病有帮助。"

第二天，老人就带着小明去山上找到了这种草，小明吃了一段时间之后，脖子真的不那么粗了。小明病好后，小花的家人也就同意了他们的婚事。至于这个草，因为到了夏天就会枯萎，再也找不到，要到明年春天才会长出来，因此，就取名为"夏枯草"。

Xia Ku Cao

There was an industrious and warm-hearted lad named Xiaoming. He and a girl named Xiaohua were lovers. But the family of Xiaohua was reluctant to marry Xiaohua to him because his neck was, as thick as a frog. Xiaoming had seen many doctors and taken many herbal medicines, but they didn't work. Therefore, he was anxious and distressed.

One day, a sallow old man with shabby clothes fell down in front of Xiaoming's house. Xiaoming carried the old man back home without hesitation and indifference, and looked after him for a period of time. When the old man got better, he noticed that Xiaoming was unhappy. He asked: "Xiaoming, why are you unhappy?"

Xiaoming told the old man: "Grandpa, my girlfriend's family is unwilling to marry her to me because of my thick neck. I have visited many physicians but none of them could work out. I am very anxious."

The old man knew Xiaoming was a good and helpful lad. He told Xiaoming: "There is a purple and worm-like grass that can solve your problem. You can find it in the mountain."

The following day the old man led Xiaoming to the mountains and found that kind of grass. After taking it for some time, Xiaoming's neck got better. Xiaoming finally married Xiaohua after his problem was completely solved. As for this grass, it withers and disappears in summer and appears in the next spring. Therefore, it is named Xia Ku Cao (Xia literally means summer; Ku literally refers to wither).

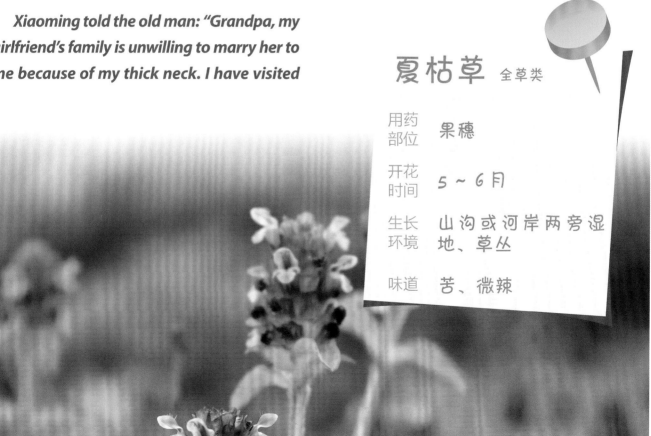

夏枯草 全草类

用药部位	果穗
开花时间	5～6月
生长环境	山沟或河岸两旁湿地、草丛
味道	苦、微辣

益母草

　　张华妈妈怀孕十月，很辛苦地生下了他。生完孩子之后，张华妈妈经常感到下腹部隐隐作痛。慢慢地张华长大了，看到妈妈总是这样的不舒服，很担忧，下定决心要治好妈妈的病。

　　张华走了很多地方找了很多医生，但是医生都没有很好的办法治疗妈妈的病，就这样又过去了十年。张华的孝心感动了上天，神仙托梦给张华，要他去山里找一种植物，这种植物长有三片叶子，叶子外形很尖，根部有一圈紫红色的小花。神仙说这个植物可以让妈妈的病慢慢好起来。

　　张华醒后，急忙赶去森林寻找，找了一天一夜，终于在离水不远，阳光充足的地方找到了这种植物。他把这种植物带回家煮汤给妈妈喝，妈妈的病果然慢慢地好了。后来人们听说了这个感人的故事，给这种植物取名为"益母草"。

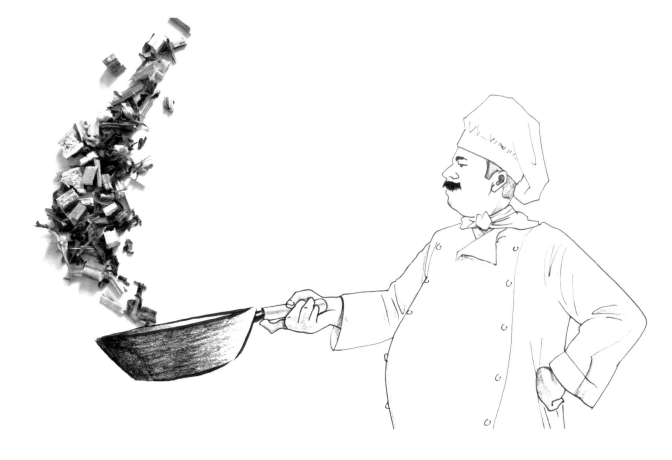

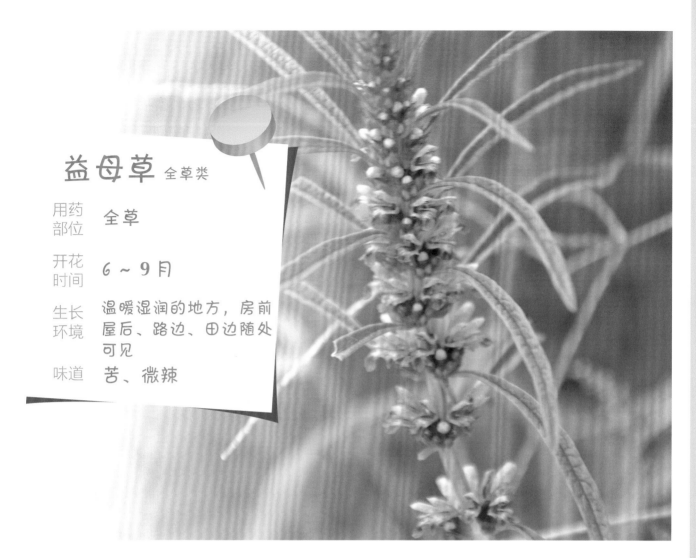

益母草 全草类

用药部位	全草
开花时间	6 ~ 9月
生长环境	温暖湿润的地方，房前屋后、路边、田边随处可见
味道	苦、微辣

Yi Mu Cao

After a 10-month pregnancy, ZhangHua was born. However, since the delivery, his mother often felt dull pain in the lower abdomen. Seeing her mother's suffering, ZhangHua was worried. Therefore, he was determined to cure his mother when he grew up.

ZhangHua visited many physicians. Although it seemed like nothing was working, he didn't give up. Ten years later, the gods in the heaven were moved by ZhangHua's filial piety. They appeared in ZhangHua's dream and told him to find a magic plant that can cure his mother. The plant had three sharp and thin leaves and at the distal end of the leaves, there were purplish red flowers.

ZhangHua hurried to the forest to find this plant after he woke up. Looking for it for a day and a night, he finally found it in a bright place near the river. He brought it home and stewed it for his mother. Gradually, his mother was recovered. Many people heard this story and were touched, so they name this herb "Yi Mu grass" (Yi literally means benefiting and Mu means mother in Chinese).

半枝莲

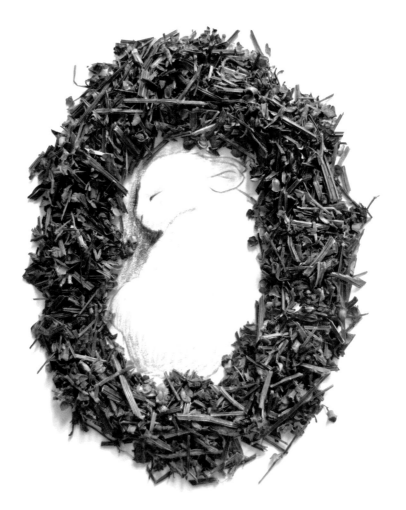

　　传说有一位老神仙来到凡间，在半山腰的一个小村庄里，听到一户人家传出很凄惨的哭泣声，神仙透过茅屋，看见几个小孩正趴在母亲身上大哭，神仙推开屋门问道："孩子们，你们的母亲怎么了？"

　　一个年长一些的孩子哭哭啼啼地答道："妈妈在山上砍柴的时候，被一条毒蛇咬伤了，已经昏迷了好久。爸爸去山下请大夫，还没回来，可是妈妈快不行了"。

　　神仙取下了随身拿着的一只莲花，将半朵莲花揉碎后涂抹在了蛇伤处，没过多久，伤口便流出许多毒汁，孩子们的妈妈也渐渐地苏醒了。孩子们高兴得跳起来："谢谢老爷爷，谢谢您救了我们妈妈。"

　　老神仙笑着摇摇头，说道："孩子们，好好照顾你们的妈妈。"说完，留下了另外半朵莲花就飞走了。突然，一阵大风将那半朵莲花吹走了，落到山野里，茂盛地生长起来，于是大家称这味中药为"半枝莲"。

Ban Zhi Lian

Legend has said that an immortal came to the earth and heard someone crying sadly in a small village halfway up the mountain. Peeking through the hut, the immortal saw several kids crying over their mother. Being curious, the immortal pushed the door open and asked: "Kids, what's the matter with your mother?"

The elder kid sobbed: "Our mum was bitten by a poisonous snake when she was cutting firewood in the mountain and has been in a coma for a time. Dad has gone to the doctor's, but mum……"

The immortal took a lotus that he was carrying around, and grinded half of it and daubed it on the wound. Soon, venom came out and the mother came to consciousness gradually. The kids jumped up happily and said: "Thank you, grandpa. Thank you for saving our mother."

The immortal shook his head and said: "kids, take good care of your mother." Then he left the other half lotus and flied away. Suddenly, a gust of wind blew the half lotus flower away, down to the wild, and it grew flourishingly, so it was called "Ban Zhi Lian" (Ban refers to half in Chinese; lian means lotus).

半枝莲 全草类

用药部位	全草
开花时间	4 ~ 7 月
生长环境	温暖湿润的地方，房前屋后、路边、田边随处可见
味道	酸

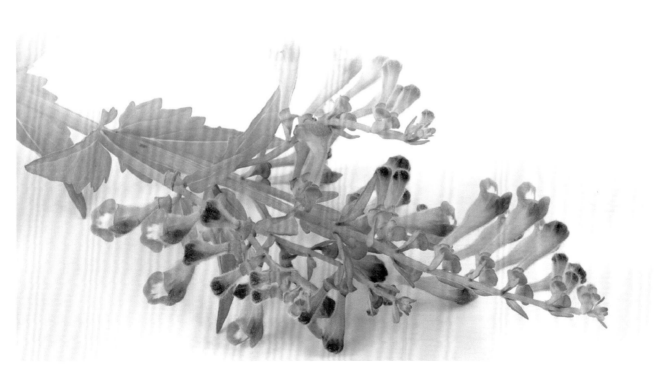

白花蛇舌草

从前，有一位很有名的医生，被请去救治一位得了重病的人。病人自觉胸闷，并且一直发热，咳出大量臭臭的痰。这位名医看了病人之后，一时间也想不出好的治疗方法，不知不觉睡着了。

梦里他遇见了一位穿着白衣服的女孩，女孩对他说："医生，那位病人是位心地善良的好人。他只要看到有人抓蛇，就会买下放生，请医生救救他。"

医生问："姑娘，我应该用什么药治好他？"

女孩说："请跟我来。"

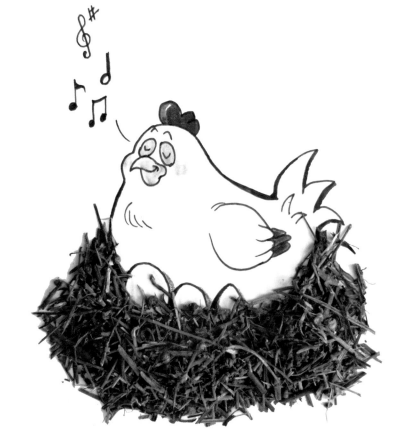

梦中他跟着女孩来到房子外面，女孩变成了一条白花蛇，蛇的舌头伸出来碰到土地上，长出来了一丛丛的小草。突然医生被附近走路的声音惊醒了。原来是病人的家属过来请医生去吃饭。

医生急忙说："先等等，请跟我来。"病人的家属跟随医生来到门外，看到了一处凹凸不平的土地上长着许多开着小白花的小草，像医生梦中看到的一样。于是医生摘了一些，告诉家属煮水给病人喝。病人喝了这种水觉得舒服了很多，接着连喝了几天，病便好了。

因为病人平时乐于行善，才得到了应有的回报。医生很感慨，他说："这些小草开在白花蛇舌头碰到的地方，就叫它'白花蛇舌草'吧。"

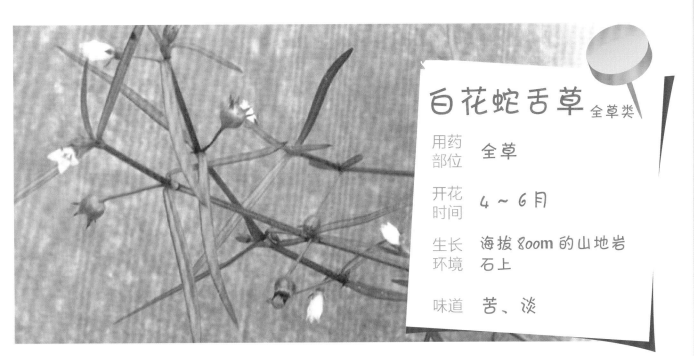

白花蛇舌草 全草类

用药部位	全草
开花时间	4～6月
生长环境	海拔800m 的山地岩石上
味道	苦、淡

Bai Hua She She Cao

Once upon a time, there was a famous doctor who was asked to treat a seriously ill man. With chest distress, fever and profuse stinky phlegm while coughing . After observing the patient, the famous doctor couldn't think of a good treatment immediately, then he fell asleep.

In the dream he met a girl in white. The girl said to him: "Doctor, the patient is a kind-hearted man. When he saw someone catching snakes, he would buy the snakes and set them free. Please help him."

The doctor asked: "Girl, which medicine can cure him?"

The girl said: "Come with me."

In the dream he followed the girl to the outside of the house. Suddenly, the girl became a long-noded pit viper (we call it white flower snake in China). The snake took out its tongue then a cluster of grass grew. He was astonished by what he saw in the dream. At this time, the doctor was awakened by the sound of walks nearby. It was the family of the patient who came over and invited the doctor to dinner.

The doctor hurriedly said: "Wait, please follow me." The doctor and the family of the patient came out, and sure enough, there was a rough place growing the little white flowers which he had seen in his dream. Then he picked some of them and told the family to boil them. The patient drank it and indeed felt better. After taking it for a few days, the patient was cured.

The doctor marveled at what the patient was rewarded for his kind-heartedness, and said: "These grasses grow in the place where the white flower snake can touch with, then let's call it Bai Hua She She Cao (which refers to white flower snake tongue grass) "

车前草

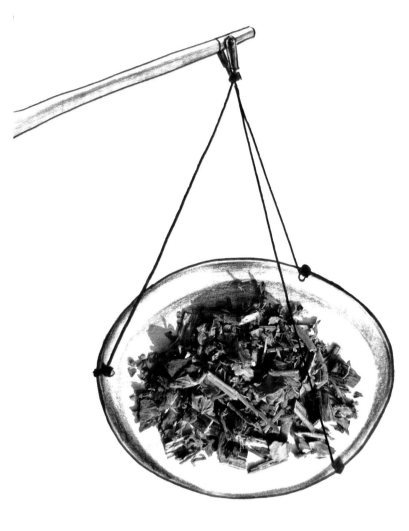

　　从前，有一位大将军打了败仗，军队被困在一个没有人烟的地方。这时正是一年中最炎热的时候，没有雨水，庄稼枯死了，粮草也吃完了。由于严重缺水，士兵和战马饿死了许多。还有很多士兵感觉肚子发胀，小便时会痛，尿的颜色发黄甚至出现血尿。不久就连战马都有了同样的症状。

　　面对这种情形，将军非常着急。有一天，马夫突然发现有几匹马尿的颜色正常了，而且精神也好了很多。马夫觉得很奇怪，就围着马仔细观察，发现这些马几天来一直吃长在战车前面的一种猪耳形状的野草。马夫猜想这些野草可能是治病良药，于是他拔了许多这种草熬水喝，连续喝了几天后，小便果然正常了。马夫急忙跑到帐篷内，把这件事情报告了将军。将军听了非常高兴，立即命令士兵们拔草煮水喝。几天后，神奇的事情发生了，所有人的病都好了。

　　将军问马夫："治病的野草长在什么地方？"

　　马夫说："就长在马车前面。"

　　将军哈哈大笑，说："好个'车前草'。"

　　从此，车前草的名字就传开了。

Che Qian Cao

车前草 全草类

用药部位	全草
开花时间	5 ~ 7 月
生长环境	房前、屋后、路边沟前，随处可见
味道	甜

Once upon a time, a great general was defeated and his army was eventually trapped in a deserted place. At that time, it was the hottest time of the year. There was no rain, no growing crops and no water. The food for soldiers and horses had been eaten up and many soldiers and horses were starved to death. A lot of soldiers, and even horses, had abdominal distension and painful urination with yellow and even reddish urine.

Facing this situation, the general was very anxious. One day, the horse-keeper noticed that some horses' urine became normal and the horses were much more energized. Surprised at this, the horse-keeper Wandered around the horses, he found the horses have been taking a kind of pig ear-shaped weeds growing before the carriages. With a guess that the horses became better because of these grasses, the horse keeper grabbed a lot of these grasses and boiled them. After drinking it for a few days, his urine also became normal. The horse keeper hurried into the tent and reported it to the general. The general was very pleased, and immediately ordered the soldiers to draw these grasses and boil them with water. A few days later, it was amazed that everyone was cured.

The general asked the horse keeper: "where do the healing weeds grow?"

The horse said "They are in front of the carriages."

The general laughed and said: "What a grass before the carriages."

From then on, the name of "a grass before the carriages" was spread.

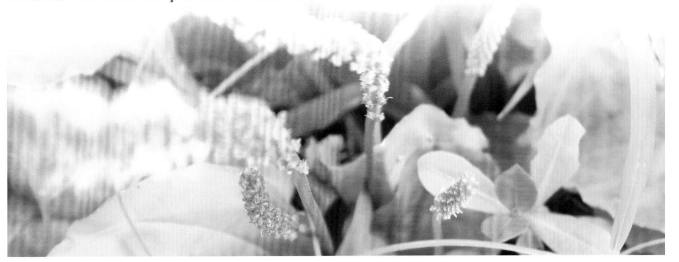

鹿衔草

古时候，皇帝带领士兵进大盘山打猎。一天，他们围截了一群梅花鹿。其中一只遍体鳞伤的小鹿在箭雨中慌乱地窜入一处灌木丛，向山脚有村庄的方向逃去。

一位正在菜园劳作的少妇，知道这个情况后，让小鹿躲进围裙救了它。数年后，这位少妇难产，肚子痛了五天五夜，仍没能产下婴儿。突然少妇听到了呦呦的鹿鸣，她清醒了过来，好像有了一些力量，回身朝床前望去，只见一只鹿正站在床前，正是当年自己救过的那只小鹿。鹿口中含着一束草，向少妇点头鸣叫。少妇取下那束草，慢慢咀嚼，很快就分娩了，母子都脱离了危险。从那以后，这则人救鹿性命，鹿感恩知报的故事，在整个大盘山区传了开来。鹿送来的那束草成了一味名贵中草药，由于当时鹿是含在口中送来的，人们就叫它"鹿衔草"。

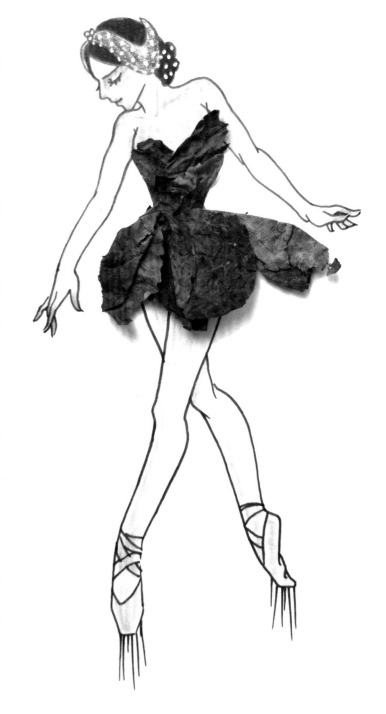

Lu Xian Cao

In ancient times, the emperor led his soldiers to hunt in the mountains. One day, they got a group of deer chased. One wounded fawn scampered around in the rains of arrows. It rushed out of a bush and ran away in the direction of the village.

A young woman, who was pulling vegetables on the farm, knew the whole story and saved the fawn by hiding it under her apron. A few years later, this young woman had not been able to deliver a baby after suffering several days' pain. Suddenly, the young woman was woken up by a fawn's crying. She felt that she had gained some strength, then she turned to the other side of the bed. She saw a deer standing beside the bed and calling her. It was the fawn that she had once saved. With a bunch of grasses in its mouth, the deer nodded to the young woman while crying. The young woman took the bunch of grasses and chewed them slowly. Soon, she delivered the baby. The mother and the baby were both out of danger. From then on, the story of the deer rewarding the woman who saved its life was spread across the whole area. The grass sent by the deer became a very expensive herbal medicine. As the deer brought the grass by biting it, people called it "deer-biting grass"(literally means 'Lu Xian Cao' in Chinese).

鹿衔草 全草类

用药部位　全草

开花时间　4～6月

生长环境　山谷溪沟旁或林下阴湿处

味道　甜中微苦

鱼腥草

有一天，一群猴子上山觅食，一只年龄最小的猴子不小心中毒了，脸肿了起来。其他猴子看见后赶忙找来了医生。

医生在山上找到了一种绿色的长着许多小花朵的小草，对小猴子的妈妈说："不要担心，把这种小草研磨了敷在脸上，就会消肿了。"

小猴子妈妈问："不用煮来喝吗？"

医生说："这种草有点鱼腥味，闻起来不舒服，所以叫'鱼腥草'。但是治疗这样的疾病最好，敷在脸上就可以。"

果然，按照医生的办法，小猴子很快就恢复了健康。

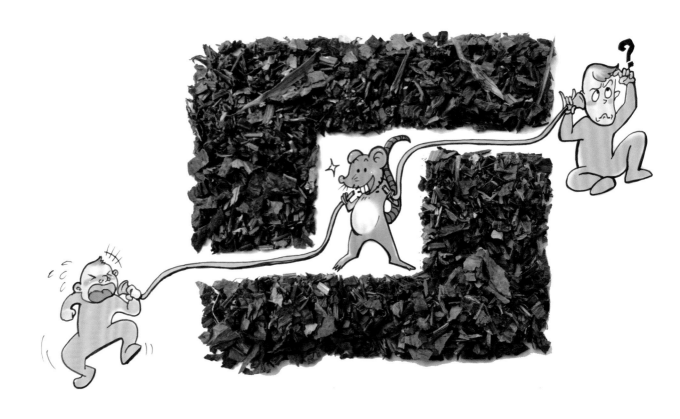

Yu Xing Cao

One day, a group of monkeys went up to the mountain to hunt for food. The youngest one was poisoned and its face became swollen. Other monkeys saw it and and rushed to invite the doctor.

The doctor found a green grass with many flowers in the mountains and gave it to the mother monkey, and said: "Don't worry. Grind the grass and apply it on the face, and it will not swollen."

The mother monkey asked: "Shouldn't I boil it for drinks?"

The doctor said: "This grass smells like fish. It was unpleasant, so we call it fish-smell grass. But it's the best method to treat a disease like this by just applying it to the face."

The mother followed the doctor's advice and the little monkey recovered soon.

鱼腥草 全草类

用药部位	带根全草
开花时间	5 ~ 6 月
生长环境	温暖潮湿的水田
味道	苦、微辣

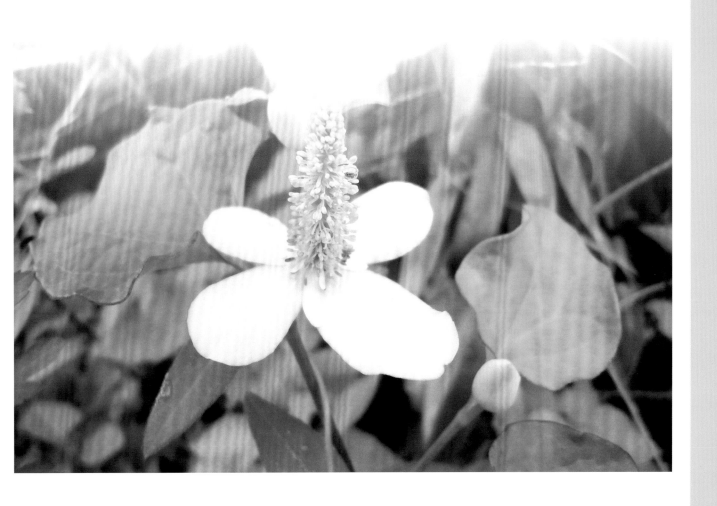

伸筋草

　　宋朝时期，一位县官为人善良，老百姓很喜欢他。冬天来了，因为缺衣少食，很多老百姓冻饿而死。为了减少这样的悲剧，县官亲自带领自己的部下给百姓们送去粮草和食物，帮助百姓渡过寒冷的冬季。可是，由于长期奔走和严寒侵袭，县官的腿出现了问题，不能够屈伸。一次送粮途中，县官双腿疼痛难忍，无法走路，众人便将他抬去找医生。

　　医生看后说："大人，您的病拖得时间太长，恐怕以后难以行走了。"

　　就在这时，一个老百姓上前说："大人的腿病是为了我们穷苦百姓才得的。我家世代在山里采药，熟知药性，我这里有一种草药，或许可以治疗大人的腿疾。"

　　说完他从背篓里面拿出一把草药，煎水给县官喝，县官喝完后觉得腿好了一些，又经过一段时间的治疗，县官的腿病彻底好了。

　　县官很感谢这位百姓，问："这个草药叫什么名字？"

　　这位百姓回答说："这个药山里人叫'山猫儿'。"

　　县官觉得这个名字不好听，于是为它取名"伸筋草"。

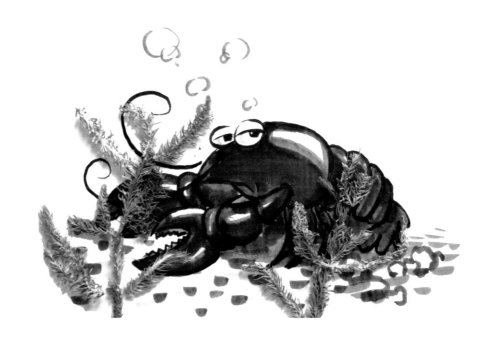

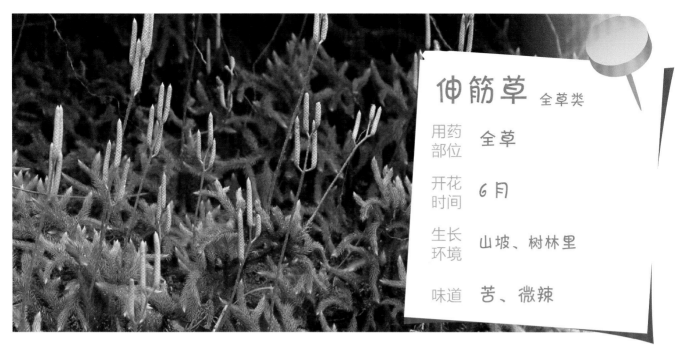

伸 筋 草 全草类

用药部位	全草
开花时间	6月
生长环境	山坡、树林里
味道	苦、微辣

Shen Jin Cao

Back to Song Dynasty, there was a kind county magistrate who was loved by the people. In the winter, many people died due to the shortage of food and clothes. In order to reduce the deaths, the county magistrate led his men to send food and clothes to the poor people and helped them survive the cold winter. However, because of the long-time busy life and the cold weather, the county magistrate had a problem in stretching and bending his legs. One day, on the way to delivering the food, the county official couldn't walk any longer because of the insufferable pains and was sent to the doctor.

the doctor said: "My Lord, you have suffered this disease for a long time. I am afraid that you aren't able to walk again."

At this time, one man in the crowd came forward and said: "The lord got this disease because of we poor people. My family has been collecting medicine in the mountains for generations. I have a kind of medicine here. Perhaps it can treat the disease."

Then he took a handful of herbs from the basket and boiled them with water. After the county magistrate took the decoction, he felt much better. After a period of treatment, the disease was treated and he could walk again.

The county magistrate was very grateful and asked: "what is the name of this herb?"
The man replied: "Well, we mountainous people call it cat in the mountain."
The county magistrate thought the name was not pleasant, so he named it "stretching grass"(literally refers to Shen Jin Cao in Chinese).

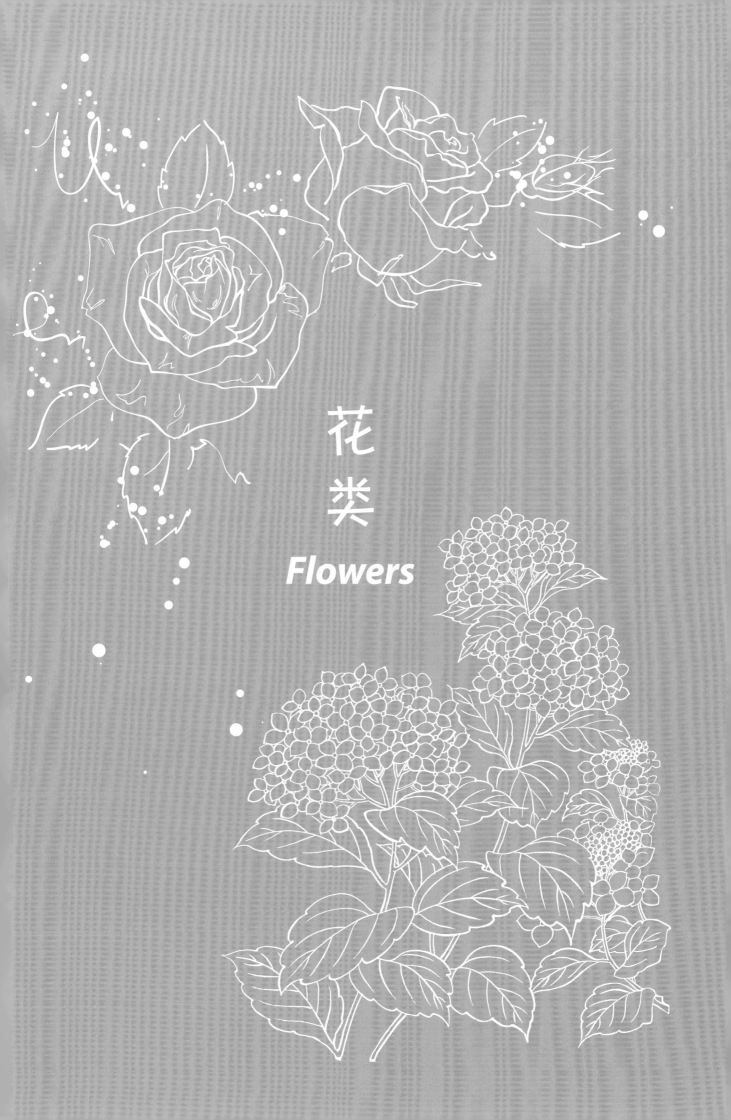

花类
Flowers

金银花

从前，一座村庄住着一对善良的夫妇，他们生了一对可爱的女儿，姐姐叫金花，妹妹叫银花。姐妹俩长得像花一样漂亮，感情也特别好。父母非常疼爱她们，乡亲、邻居们也非常喜欢这对可爱的小姐妹。

有一天，金花突然浑身发热，随后全身长满了红色的斑点。医生见后摇摇头，说："对不起，我没有办法医治这种病。"妹妹银花听到医生这么说，伤心地大哭起来。

姐姐金花流着泪对妹妹说："妹妹，你赶快离开吧，不要被我传染了。"

银花狠狠地摇了摇头，说："我不怕，我要和姐姐在一起。"银花每天都在床边照顾姐姐，可没过多久，银花也得了姐姐的这种病。姐妹俩知道没有人救得了她们，就对爸爸妈妈说："等

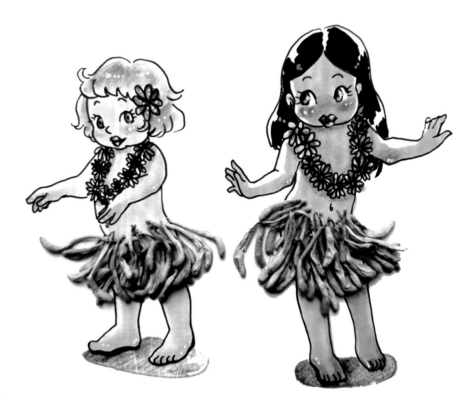

我们死后，一定要变成一棵能治我们这种病的草药，用来救治生这种病的人……"说完，姐妹俩便一起闭上眼睛，离开了这个世界。

爸爸妈妈按照她俩的临终遗言，含泪把她俩合葬在一起。

第二年的春天，她俩的坟上竟然长出一棵绿叶山藤。这棵藤苗慢慢地长大，爬满了整个坟头。到了夏天，蔓藤上长出了白色和黄色的小花朵。人们用这些小花煮水救治那些得了金花银花一样病的人们。果然，病人们身上的小红点也慢慢地消失了。大家为了感谢这对小姐妹，便把这种神奇的花叫作"金银花"。

Jin Yin Hua

Once upon a time, there lived a kind-hearted couple in the village. They gave birth to lovely twin girls. The elder girl was called Golden Flower (Jin Hua), and the younger one was named Silver Flower (Yin Hua). The girls were as beautiful as flowers, and they got along well. Their parents loved them, and the neighbors also adored the lovely little girls.

One day, Golden Flower (Jin Hua) suddenly got fever, and then red spots appeared in the whole body. The doctor shook his head and said: "Sorry. I have no way to cure this disease." The sister Silver Flower (Yin Hua) heard what the doctor said and was heartbroken with tears.

The elder sister Golden Flower (Jin Hua) shed tears to her sister and said: "Sister, you'd better leave me alone, otherwise you will be infected."

Silver Flower (Yin Hua) shook her head fiercely and said: "I'm not afraid. I will be right here with you." The Silver Flower (Yin Hua) took care of her sister by the bed every day. After a period of time, she got this disease too.

Knowing that no one could help them, the sisters told their father and mother: "We wish we can become a herb curing this disease so that those suffering from this illness will get treated..." Then the two sisters closed their eyes together and left the

金银花 花类

用药部位	花蕾或带初开的花
开花时间	4 ~ 6月
生长环境	温暖湿润的栽培土壤
味道	微苦、淡

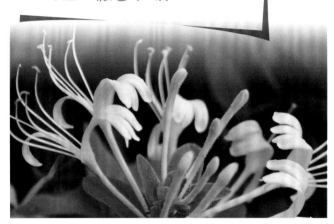

world eternally.

Their parents buried them together in tears, according to their last words.

In the spring of the following year, a green vine grew on their grave. The vine grew up slowly and wrapped the whole grave. In the summer, small white and yellow flowers grew on the vines. People used these little flowers to treat those who had the same disease with the twins. Sure enough, the sicks took the water boiled with the flowers and slowly began to get better, and the little red dots gradually disappeared. To thank the little sisters, they called this magical flower "Jin Yin Hua"(Jin means Golden and Yin refers to Silver).

野菊花

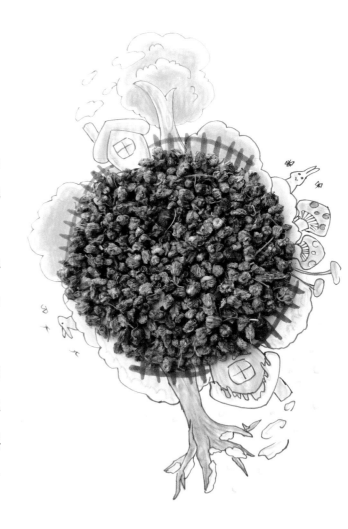

一条宽广的小河边盛开着漫山遍野的野花，小青蛙在水里游来游去。

"嗨！你怎么还在慢吞吞地游泳？洪水马上就要来了。"几只白鹅游到小青蛙身边说道。

"可是，听小麻雀说山的那边有一只蚂蚁爷爷眼睛红肿，快看不见了，他没办法搬家，可能会被洪水淹死，你说怎么办啊？"小青蛙伤感地说。

小青蛙和白鹅都觉得蚂蚁爷爷太可怜了，其中一只白鹅说："我想到一个方法可能可以救蚂蚁爷爷，治好他的眼睛，你们愿意帮他吗？"

"当然啊！可是我们要怎么做呢？"小青蛙说。

"我小时候有次眼睛肿了，爷爷摘了河边的野菊花给我吃，吃了几次眼睛就好了，这次我们也可以摘些野菊花送给蚂蚁爷爷。"

于是小伙伴行动起来，白鹅游向对岸的河边，采了野菊花，用嘴衔着游了回来，然后把野菊花交到小青蛙手里，小青蛙蹦蹦跳跳地跳过农田，把野菊花交到小麻雀的手里。小麻雀抓着野菊花飞过高山，送到蚂蚁爷爷的手里。"蚂蚁爷爷，我带来了野菊花，你赶紧吃掉，这样你的眼睛会好起来的！"

蚂蚁爷爷吃了野菊花，感觉眼睛不疼了，他缓缓睁开眼睛："真的谢谢你，小麻雀。"

"这是大家努力的结果，我们大家都希望您健健康康的。"

Ye Ju Hua

Wild flowers bloomed on the two sides of a wide river, and the little frogs swam back and forth in the water.

"Hi! You're still swimming slowly. Don't you know that the flood is on the corner?", said the white geese as they swam to the little frog.

"But I heard from the little sparrow that a grandpa ant on the other side of the mountain got red and swollen eyes. He can't move, for he can't see. He would drown in the flood. How can we do?" said the little frog sadly.

Considering the poor grandpa ant, a white goose said: "I have a way to save the grandpa ant and cure his eyes. Will you help him?"

"Of course! But how can we do?"said the little frog.

"When I was a child, I had a swollen eye. My grandpa picked wild chrysanthemum flowers along the river for me. After I took them for a few times, my eyes recovered. So we can pick some wild chrysanthemums and gave them to grandpa ant."

Then all of them were engaged into it. The white geese swam to the other side of the river to pick the small yellow wild chrysanthemum flowers with their mouths and then swam back to the frog. Then the frog carried the flowers and skipped across farmland to hand them over to the sparrow. The little sparrow held the wild chrysanthemum flowers and flied over the high mountain and gave them to grandpa ant.

"Grandpa ant, I brought you the wild chrysanthemum flowers. Eat them, and your eyes will get better!"

The grandpa ant took the wild chrysanthemum flowers, and felt the pains going away. He opened his eyes slowly and said: "Thank you so much, little sparrow."

"We are all in this, the white geese, the frog and I, and we all hope you are healthy."

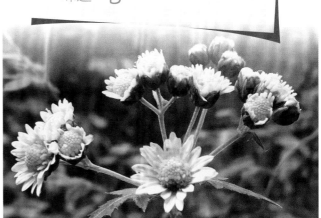

野菊花 花类

用药部位　头状花序

开花时间　9 ～ 10 月

生长环境　凉爽湿润的山坡草地、灌丛、河边水湿地，海滨盐渍地及田边、路旁

味道　苦

玫瑰花

在花王国，国王和王后有个女儿名字叫乐乐。因为脸上长了很多斑点，乐乐公主成天闷闷不乐，动不动就发脾气。国王和王后很担心公主，于是公告天下，谁可以让公主快乐起来，就可以实现他的一个愿望。

有一位年轻的小伙子来到国王面前，说："国王，我有一个办法可以让公主快乐起来。"

国王一听，非常高兴："你快说，什么办法？"

小伙子说："只要摘一些您花园里面独有的玫瑰花，每日泡水让公主服用，公主会渐渐快乐起来的。"

国王立刻依法照做。过了几个月，公主变得温和有礼，皮肤也渐渐变得红润，斑点少了很多，公主终于露出了快乐的微笑。国王非常高兴，请来那位小伙子问："感谢你让公主重新快乐起来，那么你有什么愿望吗？"

小伙子答道："我只想国王把玫瑰花的种子分给更多有需要的人。"

国王很羞愧地说道："美好的事物应该大家一起分享，这样才会更快乐，更有价值！"

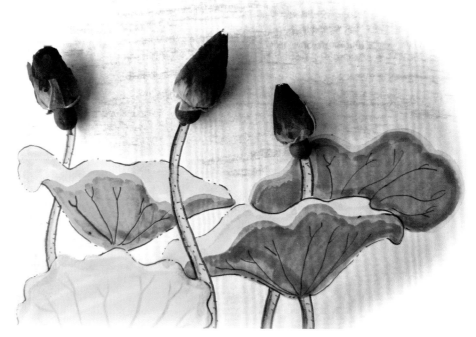

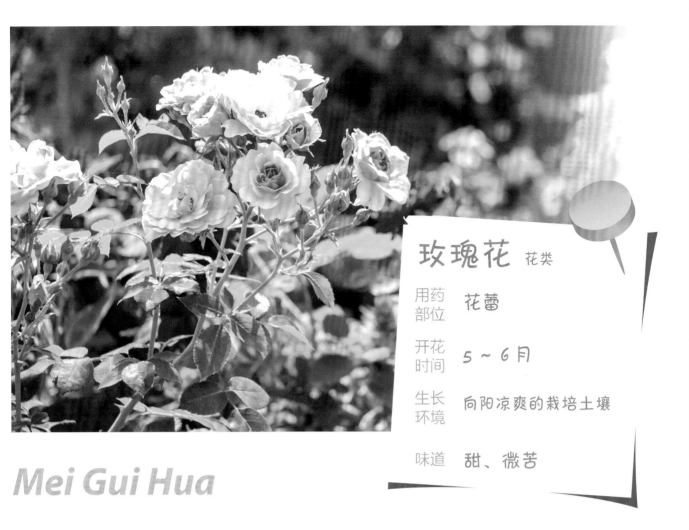

玫瑰花 花类

用药部位	花蕾
开花时间	5 ~ 6月
生长环境	向阳凉爽的栽培土壤
味道	甜、微苦

Mei Gui Hua

In the flower kingdom, the king and the queen had a daughter named Le Le (literally means happy in Chinese). As there were many speckles on her face, the princess was not happy at all. Moreover, she was rather irritable. The king and the queen were very worried about this. So they issued an announcement that the king and the queen would like to help the one who can make the princess happy make one of his wishes come true.

A young lad came to the king and said, "My king, I have a way to make the princess happy."

The king was very pleased and said: "what are you going to do?"

The young man said: "Take some of the roses in your garden, boil them and let the princess take it every day,and she will be happy."

The king immediately followed the lad's advice. After a few months, the princess became gentle in temper with reddish skin and less speckles. A smile finally showed up on the face of the princess. The king was very glad and asked the young man: "The princess is happy now. So, do you have any wishes?"

The young man replied, "Yes, I just want the king to give the seeds of the roses to more people who need them."

Being ashamed, the king said: "Beautiful things should be shared together. In this way, they will be happier and more valuable."

紫花地丁

从前，有一对兄弟俩相依为命，感情十分深厚。有一天，弟弟手指突然疼痛难忍，哥哥十分着急，于是带着弟弟去找医生，但是医生也毫无办法。兄弟俩疲惫地走回家，太阳落山了，霞光照在山坡上。哥哥指着远处的花对弟弟说："弟弟，你看紫色的花很漂亮，我们去看看吧。"

弟弟说："好的，我也想去看看。"

兄弟俩走过去，看到绿绿的草地里开着紫色的花朵。他们躺了下来，把紫色的花都压碎了。弟弟的手指无意间碰到了压碎的液体，觉得手指没有那么疼了。

弟弟说："哥哥，我的手指头凉凉的，不那么疼了。"

他们高兴地采了一些花带回家，捣烂敷在手指头上，并把剩下的煮水喝了。

第二天，弟弟手指一点都不疼，也不肿了，几天后，竟奇迹般地痊愈了。哥哥说："弟弟，这紫色的花开在绿绿的草地上，我们叫它'紫花地丁'吧。"

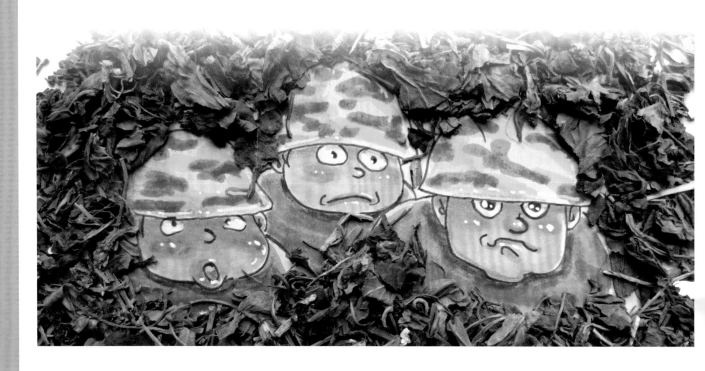

Zi Hua Di Ding

Once upon a time, there were two brothers who lived together, and they got along well. One day, the younger brother suddenly got unbearable pains in his fingers. His brother was very anxious and visited the doctor with his young brother, but there was nothing the doctor could do. So they walked home wearily. At this time, the sun set, and the sunlight shone on the hillside. Pointing to the flowers in the distance, the elder boy said: "Brother, the purple flowers there are beautiful, let's go and have a look."

The younger brother said: "Ok, I want to see it, too."

The two brothers walked over. They looked at the green grassland and the purple flowers, they laid down and accidentally crushed the purple flowers. The younger brother touched the juices unintentionally. Suddenly he felt less pain.

"My brother," said the younger brother, "my fingers are cool and not so painful."

They happily picked some flowers and took them home. They mashed some flowers and applied them on the fingers, and then drank the rest with the boiled water.

The next day, the younger brother's finger did not hurt at all, and it was not swollen. A few days later, it was cured miraculously. "Brother," said the elder one, "the purple flowers grow on the green grass. Let's call it Zi Hua Di Ding (which literally means purple flowers on the land in Chinese)."

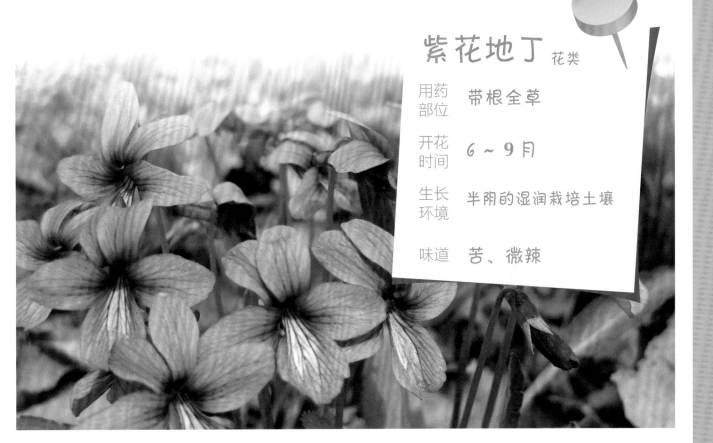

紫花地丁 花类

用药部位	带根全草
开花时间	6 ~ 9月
生长环境	半阴的湿润栽培土壤
味道	苦、微辣

栀子花

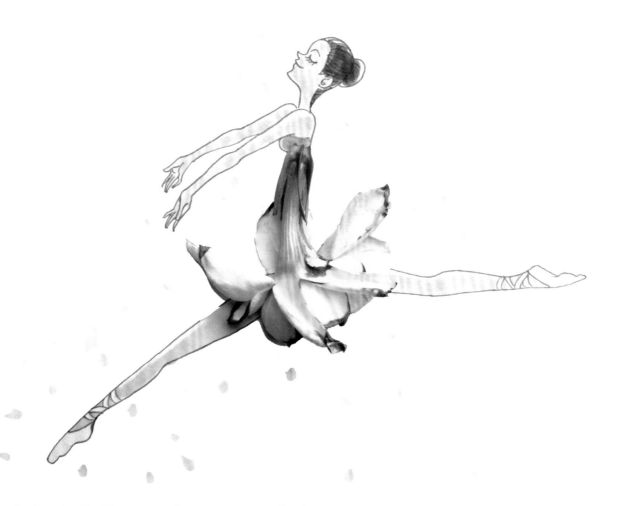

　　小月和爷爷上山采药，山非常高，路也很难走。一不小心，小月摔了一跤，脚面肿了起来，而且很痛。爷爷赶紧采了一大把栀子花，扶着小月回了家。小月问爷爷："爷爷，您拿栀子花是做什么？"

　　爷爷回答说："这是给你治脚伤的。"

　　小月很好奇，她看着爷爷把栀子花捣碎，然后打了一个鸡蛋，用蛋清和捣碎的栀子花调成糊状，敷在小月的脚背上。

　　小月对爷爷说："爷爷，这草药敷到脚上凉凉的，很舒服，也没有那么痛了。"

　　爷爷笑了，说："这栀子花也是一味中药哦。"

　　小月看着桌上美丽的白色的栀子花，心想："原来这么漂亮的栀子花，也可以用作中药治病呀。"

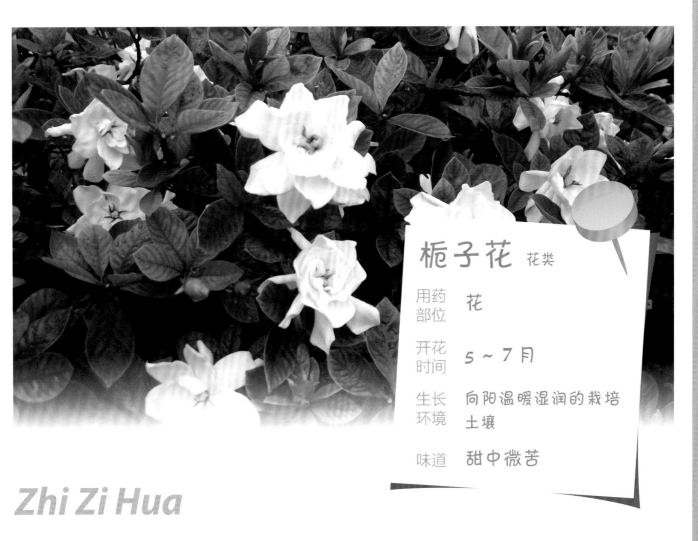

栀子花 花类

用药部位	花
开花时间	5 ~ 7 月
生长环境	向阳温暖湿润的栽培土壤
味道	甜中微苦

Zhi Zi Hua

One day, Xiaoyue and her grandpa went to the mountains to pick herbal medicines. The mountain was very high, and it was a difficult climb. Carelessly, Xiaoyue had a fall and her feet were swollen and painful. Grandpa hurried to pick a bunch of gardenia flowers, and supported Xiaoyue back home. Xiaoyue asked: "Grandpa, what do you do with gardenia flowers?"

Grandpa answered: "They are to treat your feet."

Being curious, Xiaoyue watched her grandfather pound the gardenia and mix it with egg white. After the mixture was stirred into a paste, grandpa applied it to Xiaoyue's feet.

"Grandpa," she said to grandfather, "my feet feel cool and comfortable, and they are not so painful."

Grandpa smiled and said: "Gardenia flower is also a Chinese herb."

Looking at the beautiful white gardenia flowers on the table, Xiaoyue thought: "It turns out that these beautiful gardenia flower can also be used as Chinese medicine."

七叶一枝花

　　很久以前，天目山上住着一个青年叫沈见山，靠砍柴为生。一天，他在砍柴时，草丛中忽然窜出一条毒蛇，他还没来得及躲避，小腿就被蛇狠狠咬了一口。不一会儿，他就昏迷在地，不省人事。说来也巧，天上的七仙女正好脚踏彩云来天目山天池洗澡，看到了昏倒的沈见山，便动了恻隐之心，她们将他围成一圈，取出随身携带的罗帕盖在他的伤口四周。更巧的是，王母娘娘这时也驾祥云到此，她随手拔下头上的碧玉簪，放在七块罗帕的中央。因为罗帕和碧玉簪的仙气，伤口处的蛇毒很快就消散了，沈见山徐徐醒来。一瞬间，罗帕和碧玉簪一起落在了地上，变成了七片翠叶托着一朵金花的野草。沈见山惊呆了，仿佛刚做了一场梦，又看看自己的小腿，也没有伤痕。他想是这美丽的野草救了自己，于是给它取名为"七叶一枝花"。后来村民们每遇有蛇咬伤患者，就采挖此药救治伤者。

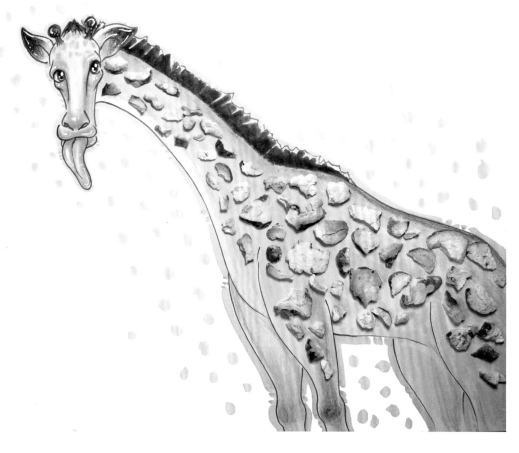

Qi Ye Yi Zhi Hua

Once upon a time, there was a young man named Shen Jianshan who lived in Tian Mu mountain. He made a living cutting firewood. One day, while he was cutting firewood, a poisonous snake suddenly appeared in the grass. His lower leg was bitten by the snake before he could avoid it. Soon he became unconscious and fell down. Luckily, the seven fairies who lived in the heaven happened to take a ride by colorful clouds to the heaven pool on the Tian Mu Mountain for a bath. They saw Shen lying on the ground and wanted to help him, so they circled around him and covered the wound by the handkerchiefs that they always carry with them. Coincidentally, the queen of the heaven also drove here by the auspicious cloud. She took off the green jade hairpin and put it in the center of the handkerchiefs. The magic qi from the handkerchiefs and green jade hairpin healed the wound and the venom quickly dissipated. Later, Shen came to consciousness. A moment after he woke up, the handkerchiefs and green jade hairpin dropped on the ground, and instantly became a grass with seven green leaves bearing a golden flower. He was shocked as if he had just had a dream. Then he looked at his leg and there was no scar. He thought it was this beautiful weed that saved him, and named it "a flower with seven leaves". Later, for every snake bite, the villagers would collect and pick this flower for treatment and every time it worked.

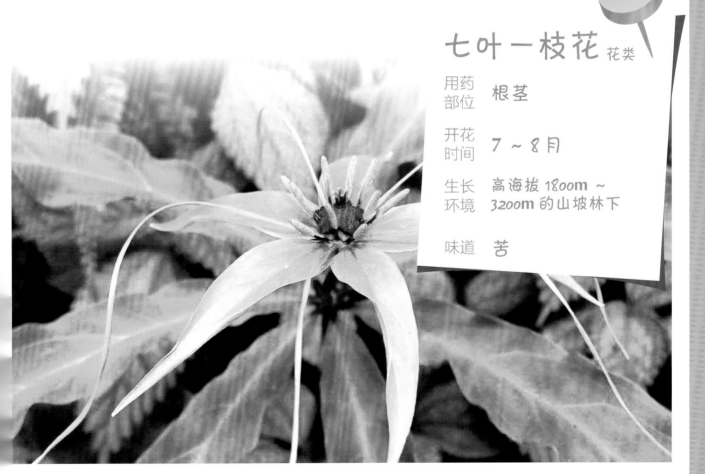

七叶一枝花 花类

用药部位	根茎
开花时间	7 ~ 8月
生长环境	高海拔 1800m ~ 3200m 的山坡林下
味道	苦

槐花

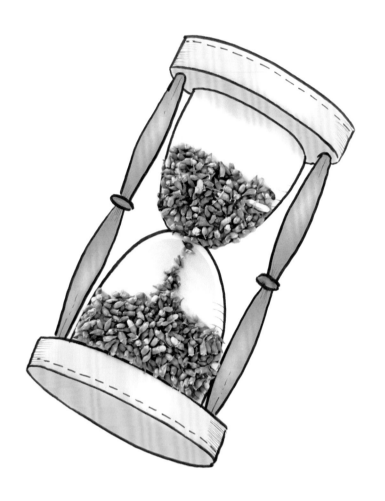

　　宋代有位书生家里栽种着一棵槐树，到了春天，一串串洁白的槐花挂满枝头，空气中弥漫着淡淡的清香，书生十分喜爱这样的场景。

　　有一年，正是槐花开放的季节，书生的舌头突然不停地出血，几个医生看过都不知道是什么病，更找不到解除病痛的办法。书生很着急，慕名找到当地名医赵瑜，赵瑜看到书生家里槐树开满槐花，兴奋地对他说，"你家的槐花正是治疗你这个病的良药呀！"书生非常吃惊，没想到美丽的槐花还有这样的功效！书生按照赵瑜的建议把槐花摘下来，磨成细细的粉末敷在舌头上，马上觉得舒服多了。坚持敷了几天后，他的舌头就不再出血了。

　　书生将槐花治病的故事告诉了周围的邻居，大家从此都知道了槐花有止血的功效。

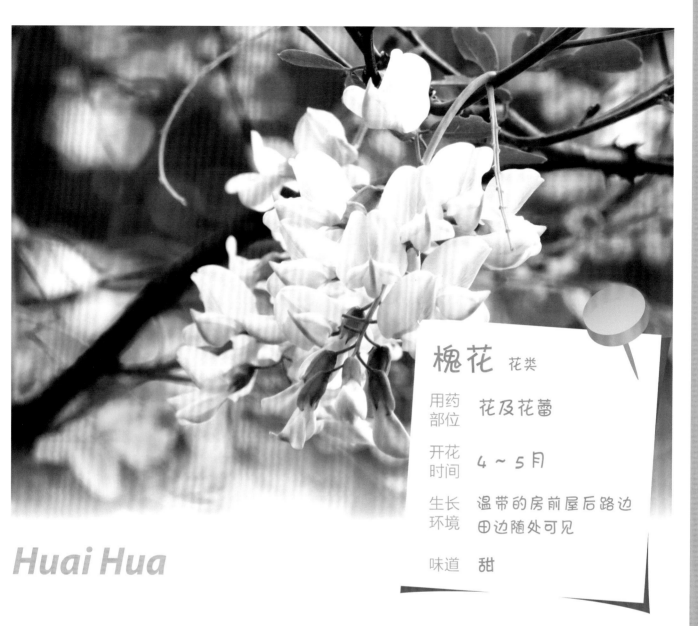

槐花 花类

用药部位	花及花蕾
开花时间	4～5月
生长环境	温带的房前屋后路边田边随处可见
味道	甜

Huai Hua

In song dynasty, there was a scholar who planted a pagoda tree in his garden. Every spring, strings of white flowers hung on the branches, filling the air with light fragrance. He loved it very much.

One year at the time when the flowers bloom, the scholar's tongue started bleeding. Several doctors didn't know what the disease was or how to deal with it. After examination, Zhao Yu, a famous doctor, noticed the pagoda tree full of flowers, and said to him excitedly: "Your pagoda tree flower is the effective medicine to cure your disease!" Being surprised at the effective role of beautiful pagoda tree flower, the scholar followed the doctor's advice. After picking off the flowers, he grinding them into fine powder and applied it to the tongue, and he felt much better at once. Keeping the treatment for a few days, his tongue stopped bleeding.

He told the neighbors that the pagoda tree flower can treat disease. Since then, everyone knew that the pagoda tree flower could stop bleeding.

丁香花

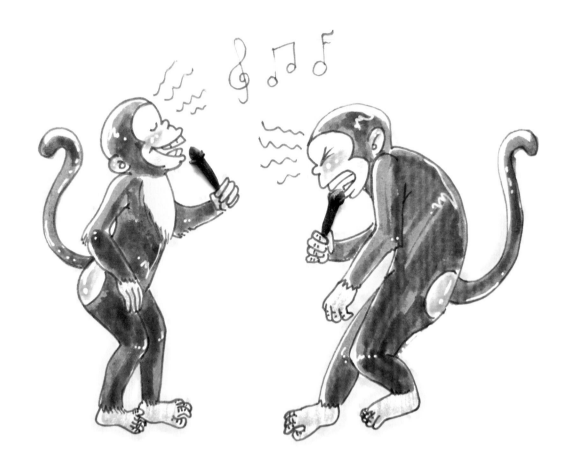

　　古代一个皇帝爱吃生冷的食物。一个酷暑的夜晚，喝完冰粥的皇帝突然感觉肚子又胀又痛，上吐下泻，特别难受。太医看过也找不到好办法，只有张榜寻找民间名医。不久，一名乞丐揭榜入宫，诊过脉后对皇帝说："皇上喜欢吃生冷的食物，伤到脾胃，用丁香等鲜花制成香袋挂在床边可以缓解症状。"

　　皇帝马上派人采集新鲜的丁香花，晒干，制成香囊挂在床边，清新的香味让皇帝感到很舒服。几天后，皇帝的症状就消失了。他很高兴，想要奖赏那名乞丐，于是派人在京城四处寻找，却怎么也找不到了。当晚，皇帝梦见乞丐原来是八仙之一的采药仙人蓝采和所变。第二天皇帝就让太医将丁香的功效和用法记下，并称丁香为神仙赐予的药。丁香的药用价值从此流传下来。

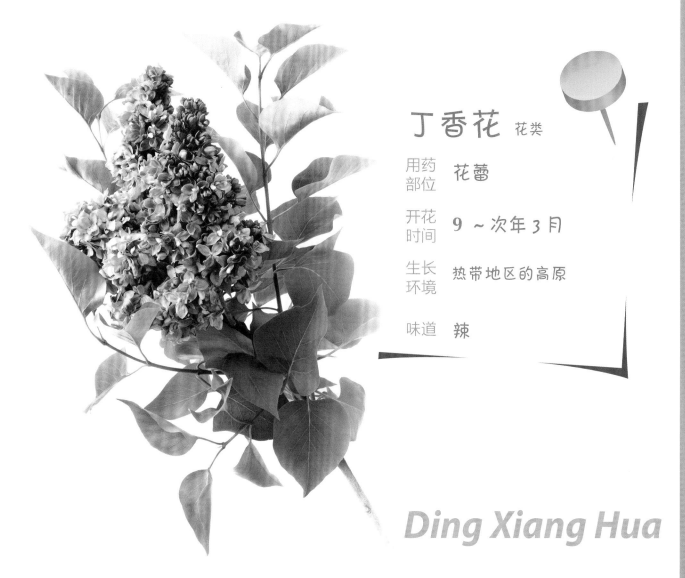

丁香花 花类

用药部位	花蕾
开花时间	9 ~ 次年 3 月
生长环境	热带地区的高原
味道	辣

Ding Xiang Hua

An ancient emperor loved to eat raw and cold food. On a hot summer night, after eating some icy porridge, the emperor suddenly had abdominal distension and pains with vomiting and diarrhea. The imperial physicians could not find a good treatment after examining the emperor, so they had to put up an imperial notice to hunt for good folk physicians. After Seeing the notice, a beggar took off the notice and went into the imperial court. He said: "The emperor likes to eat raw and cold food, which hurts his spleen and stomach. He can make a sachet of lilac flowers and hang it on the bed."

The emperor immediately sent someone to gather fresh lilacs and dried them to make a sachet. The fresh fragrance made the emperor feel very comfortable. A few days later, the symptoms disappeared. The emperor was so happy that he wanted to reward the beggar, so he sent someone to look for him. However, the beggar magically disappeared. That night, the emperor dreamed of the beggar. It turned out that the beggar was Lan Caihe, the herbal immortal, one of the eight immortals. The next day, the emperor ordered the imperial physician to write down the effects and uses of lilac and called it the medicine given by the immortal. Since then, the therapeutic effects of lilac have come down.

旋覆花

天庭花园中的花儿们都有妖艳貌美的外表，喜欢争奇斗艳。特别是在一年一度的斗花大会上更是各出奇招，都想要吸引花管家的注意，以此提高在花园中的地位，争得"花神"的称号。

只有旋覆花，开着淡黄色的小花，不愿看他人的脸色行事，从不参与攀比。因此，每次斗花大会中旋覆花都会被忽略，地位日益下降。

一年一度的斗花大会又要开始了，大家都在积极打理自己的花瓣，热火朝天地讨论，旋覆花却没什么反应。同伴都看不下去，纷纷劝旋覆花应该好好打扮，在管家面前好好表现自己，才能获得更高的地位。旋覆花却说："我只要有自己的工作和安稳的生活就满足了，并不想争花神。"这句话被恰巧经过的管家听到了。

后来封神的结果出来，管家成全了旋覆花，让它显示出独特的性能，这正符合旋覆花的想法，它十分高兴，表示一定勤勤恳恳完成工作，不辜负管家的信任。这就是"诸花皆升，旋覆独降"的传说。而旋覆花确实一直低调不争坚守岗位，是功效独特又不可或缺的一种花，在花园中独享自己一方天地。

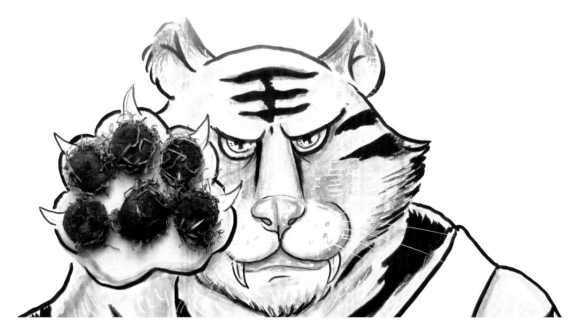

Xuan Fu Hua

With attractive appearances, all the flowers in the heaven garden like to contend in beauty and fascination. Especially at the annual flower show, all of them are trying to draw the attention of the housekeepers so as to improve their position in the garden and win the title of flower god.

However, only the little yellow Xuan Fu Hua, the inula flower, didn't want to compete in the hower show. Being low profile, Xuan Fu Hua has been neglected in every flower show and become less and less important.

When the year's flower show was around corner. Every other flower was busy arranging its petals and discussing it enthusiastically. However, Xuan Fu Hua didn't join them. The others persuaded Xuan Fu Hua to dress up and present in front of the housekeeper for higher status. But Xuan Fu Hua said: "I am satisfied with my work. I just want to lead a stable life, and I don't want to fight for the flower god." The housekeeper who happened to be passing by heard what it said and was aware of how the flower felt.

Later, the result of the competition came out. The housekeeper was fulfilled what Xuan Fu Hua dreamed of——just be itself and be unique. Xuan Fu Hua was very happy and said that it would be diligent in work and wouldn't disappoint the housekeeper. This is the story of "all flowers rising but Xuan Fu Hua sinking". Being low profile and with no desire to compete, Xuan Fu Hua stuck to its post and enjoyed itself in the garden with unique effects and an indispensable role.

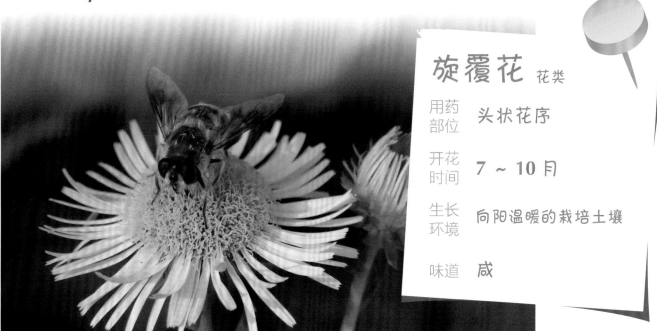

旋覆花 花类

用药部位　头状花序

开花时间　7 ~ 10 月

生长环境　向阳温暖的栽培土壤

味道　咸

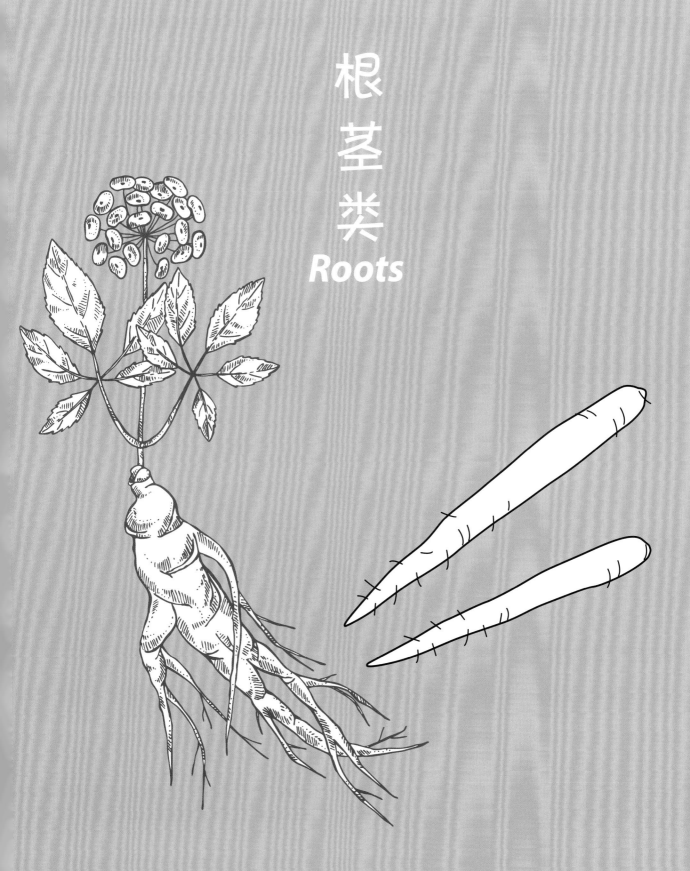

根
茎
类
Roots

山药

在一个缺衣少食的年代，有一对心肠很坏的夫妇，他们没有孝心，总盼着年老的婆婆早点过世，每天只给婆婆吃一碗稀粥。一段时间以后，婆婆浑身无力，卧床不起。这件事儿让村里的一个老中医知道了，他将计就计，想出了一个主意。他把这对夫妇叫来，给了他们一种药粉说："把这个药粉混在粥里，保证你们家老婆婆活不过一百天。"这对夫妇回去后就照这个方法煮了粥天天给老婆婆吃。没想到，十天后，老婆婆竟然能够起床活动了，三个月后老人养得白白胖胖。婆婆身体好了，在村里边逢人就夸儿子媳妇对她好。这对夫妇此时才知道老中医的良苦用心，想起以前的所作所为，真是羞愧难当。老中医趁此机会告诉他们，那个药粉就是山药做的。经过这番教导，这一对不孝夫妇变成了一对孝顺的夫妇，这个故事已成为一段佳话流传至今。

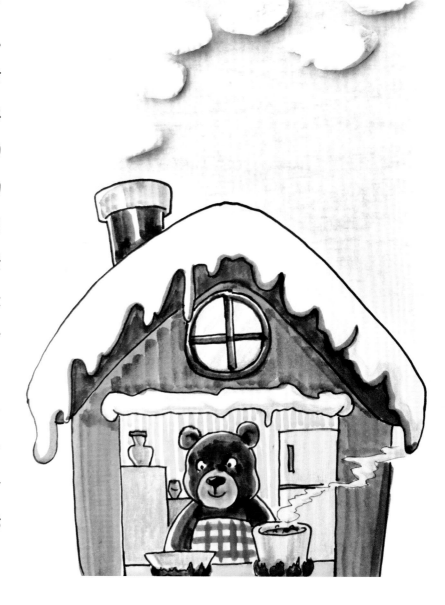

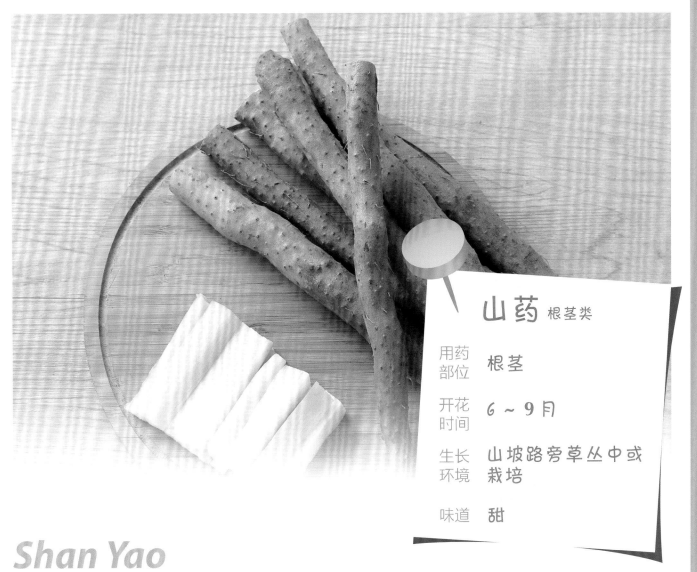

山药 根茎类

用药 部位	根茎
开花 时间	6 ~ 9月
生长 环境	山坡路旁草丛中或 栽培
味道	甜

Shan Yao

In a period of food,clothing shortage, there was a bad couple who had no filial piety. They expected their old mother to die early. Therefore, they only fed her a bowl of thin porridge every day. After a period of time, the mother was too weak to stand up. She lay in bed all day. An old physician knew about this and he came up with an idea. He called up the couple and gave them a bag of powder, he said "mix this powder with the porridge and I will make sure that the old mother will die within one hundred days." The couple went back and followed what the physician said. They put the powder in the porridge and fed their mother every day. Unexpectedly, ten days later, the mother could get up; three months later, the old mother became strong. In good health, the mother praised everyone she met at the village that her son and daughter-in-law were kind-hearted. At this time, the couple knew what the physician was up to and felt that it was a shame for what they did to their mother before. The old physician took the opportunity to tell the couple that the powder was made of Chinese yam. Learning from this lesson, the unfilial couple became a filial one, and the story was passed on from generation to generation.

地黄

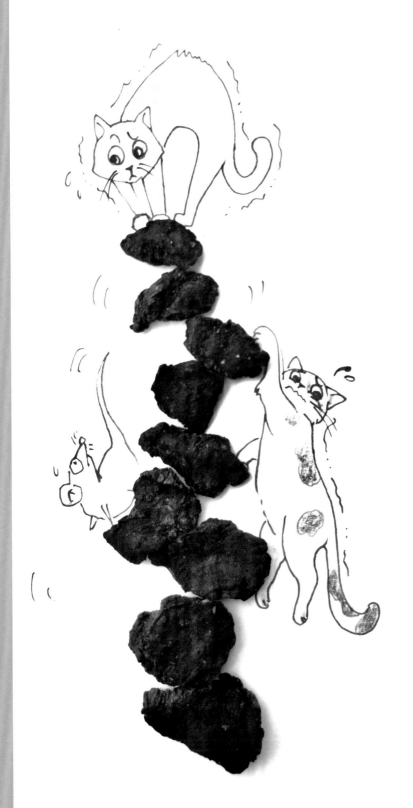

唐朝时期，有一年，黄河的中下游发生瘟疫，疾病传播速度很快，很多老百姓失去了生命。县太爷非常忧虑，来到神农山的药王庙祈求老天保佑。突然，药王庙的外边来了一个人，送给县太爷一块植物的根，送药人将这个药草称为"地皇"，意思是皇天赐药，并告诉他神农山北边的洼地里有许多这种药草，用它榨汁给病人服用就能治病。县太爷听了非常高兴，立即安排人手上山采挖，老百姓吃了药汁后果然很快痊愈了。瘟疫过后，百姓们把它引种到自家农田里种植，并且流传到全国各地。因为它的颜色发黄，百姓便把地皇叫作"地黄"了。

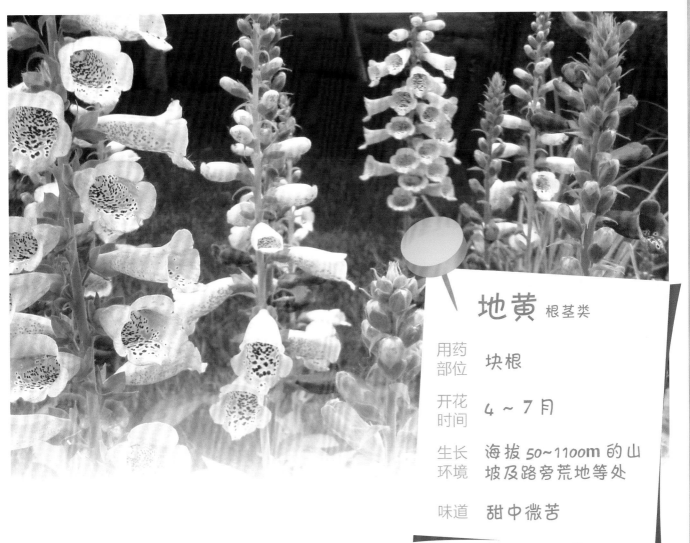

地黄 根茎类

用药部位	块根
开花时间	4 ~ 7 月
生长环境	海拔 50~1100m 的山坡及路旁荒地等处
味道	甜中微苦

Di Huang

In Tang Dynasty, plague occurred in the middle and lower reaches of the Yellow River. It spread quickly and took many lives. Being extremely anxious, the county official came to the temple of Yao Wang (Herb King) in Shen Nong Mountain for praying. At this time, a man came into the temple and sent a lump of root to the official. The man called this root Di Huang (地皇 , literally means the herb sent by the imperial god). He told the official that this herb grew profusely in the low-lying land in the north of Shen Nong Mountain. Mill the root and let the patient take the juice, and they would recover soon. Hearing this, the official was very happy. He immediately arranged for men to dig these plants. After taking the juices, the patients recovered soon. After the plague, people started to plant this herb and later the herb was spread to the whole country. Because the root is yellow, people also call it Di Huang (地黄 ; Huang means yellow).

当归

　　四川是一个盛产药材的地方，当地有一户人家靠采药、卖药为生。家里的年轻男子阿明新婚不久，就去山上采药。谁知竟一去不返，一晃三年过去了，媳妇等了三年，失去了信心，只好改嫁。谁知一年后，丈夫阿明回来了，家里媳妇却不见了，他四处寻找，终于找到了媳妇的新家。媳妇向阿明哭诉："三年当归你不归，片纸只字也不回，如今我已错嫁人，心如刀割真后悔。"阿明也懊悔自己没有按时回来，得知媳妇因为日夜思念他而得了气血亏损的妇科疾病，于是把采集的草药拿去给媳妇治病。后来，这种草药成为治疗妇科疾病的良药。后人为汲取"当归不归，娇妻改嫁"的惨痛教训，便把这个草药叫作"当归"。

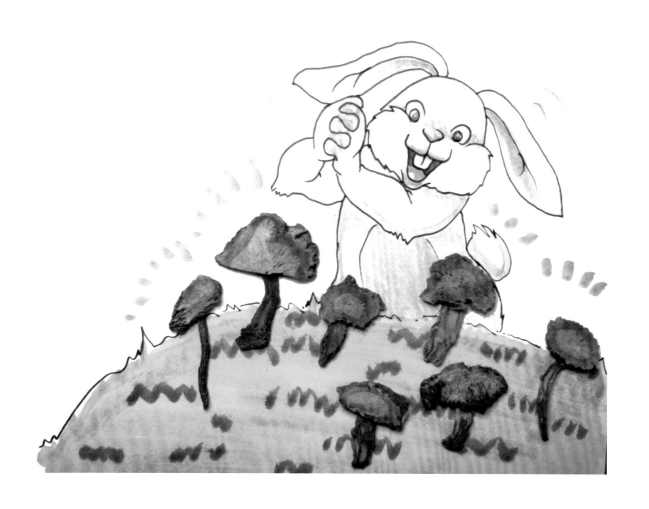

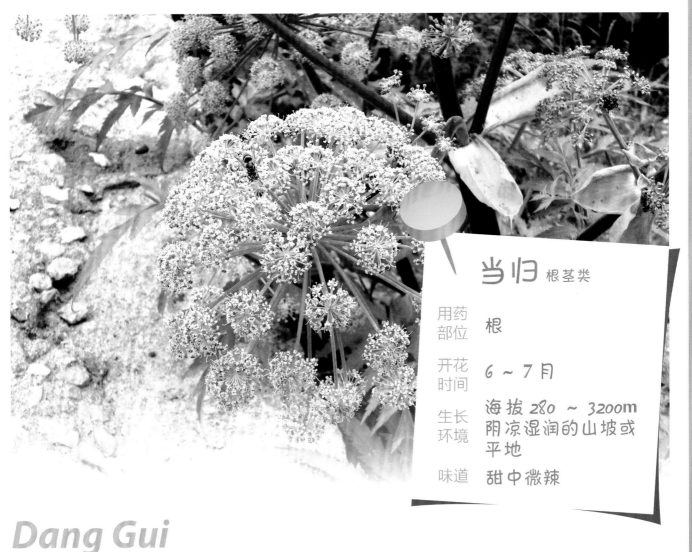

当归 根茎类

用药部位	根
开花时间	6 ~ 7 月
生长环境	海拔 280 ~ 3200m 阴凉湿润的山坡或平地
味道	甜中微辣

Dang Gui

Sichuan province is a place rich in medicinal materials. There was a family that lived on picking herbal medicines and selling them to drug stores for living materials. One day, A Ming, a young man of this family, got married. Shortly after his wedding, he went to the mountains to pick herbs. but he never returned. After three years, there was still no word from him. His wife was depressed and sad because she missed her husband for a long time. Waiting waited for three years, the wife lost confidence in his return, so she remarried. However, one year after her remarriage, her ex-husband, A Ming returned, but the wife was gone. After searching, he finally found her new home. The wife cried to A Ming: "For three years, you didn't come back. I didn't even get a word from you. Now I am already married another man. Now my heart is torn with grief and regret." A Ming also regretted that he did not return on time. Learning that his wife was sick because she missed him day and night, A Ming sent the herbs he picked to his wife for treatment. Unexpectedly, these herbs cured her gynecological diseases. Later, this herb was a fine medicine for gynecological diseases. In order to learn the painful lessons of "the beautiful wife's remarriage due to his delayed return", the herb is called "Dang Gui (当归 ; which mean that you should return)".

红景天

相传，天上有三位仙女经常到长白山天池中沐浴。一天，三姐妹在小天池嬉戏时，从远方飞来一只美丽的小鸟，将口中衔的一枚红果吐在小妹佛库伦的衣衫之上。三姐妹上岸后，佛库伦发现了这枚红果，便将其含于口中，不料一不小心将这枚红果吃到了肚子里。准备飞回天宫的时候，小妹发现自己不能飞了，只好将刚刚吃红果的事告诉两位姐姐。两位仙女回天宫向父母诉说此事，父母也毫无办法。这样佛库伦就只好留在长白山下的一个古洞居住。不久，佛库伦产下一名男婴，取名阿骨打。天上的父母日夜挂念着佛库伦，为了使她在人间保持健康的身体和强壮的体力，派佛库伦的两位姐姐把景天仙草的种子带到长白山，让佛库伦种在古洞四周，经常采挖食用，以强筋健骨，增加身心的活力。就这样，佛库伦凭着景天仙草的神力，将阿骨打抚养长大。长大后的阿骨打英姿神武，勇猛彪悍。最终成为部落首领，并逐步统一了长白山的各个部落，建立了金国，成为金国的国王，而那个红色的景天仙草也成了保护人民健康的良药。

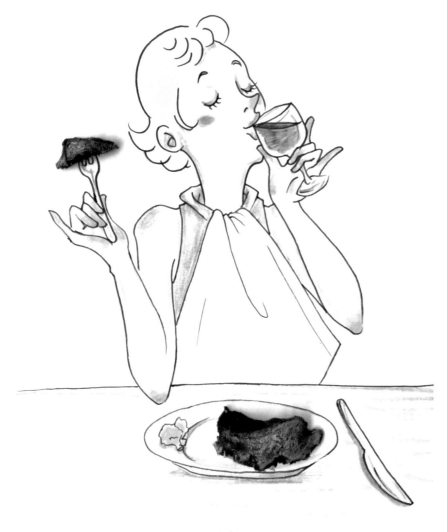

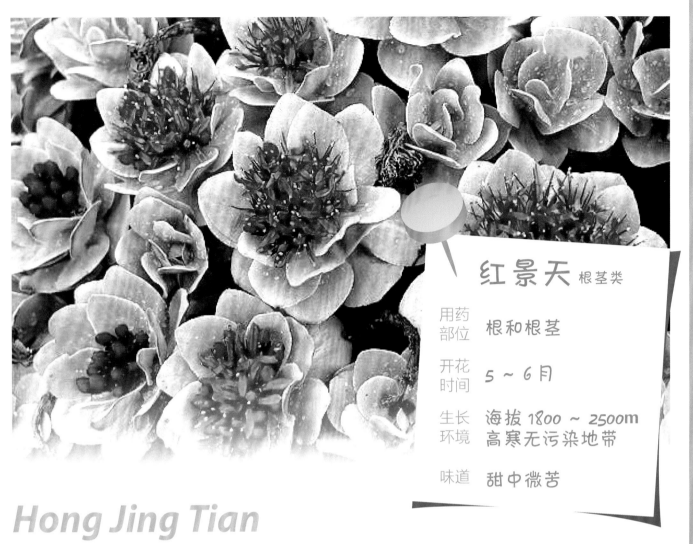

红景天 根茎类

用药部位	根和根茎
开花时间	5 ~ 6 月
生长环境	海拔 1800 ~ 2500m 高寒无污染地带
味道	甜中微苦

Hong Jing Tian

 Legend has it that three fairies often bathed in the Heaven Pool of Chang Bai Mountain. One day, when the three sisters were playing in the Heaven Pool, a beautiful bird came from afar and spat a red fruit to Fo Kulun's clothes, the youngest sister. When the three sisters went ashore, Fo Kulun found the red fruit and put it in her mouth. Accidentally, she swallowed it. When they were ready to fly back to the heaven palace, the youngest sister found that she was unable to fly. So she told two sisters about the red fruit that she had taken. The two fairies went back to the heaven and told this to their parents. However, they also didn't have a better solution. So Fo Kulun had to stay in an ancient cave in Chang Bai Mountain. Shortly afterwards, Fo Kulun gave birth to a baby boy named Aguda. The parents in the heaven missed Fo Kulun so much. In order to keep the youngest daughter healthy and strong on the earth, they sent the other two daughters to bring the seeds of a fairy grass named Jing Tian to Chang Bai Mountain and asked Fo Kulun to plant them near the cave for food. In this way, with the magic power of the fairy grass, Fo Kulun raised her son. When the boy grew up, he became tall and strong. As he fought bravely, he became a leader of a tribe. Gradually, he united several tribes of Chang Bai Mountain, founded the Jin dynasty and became the king. As for the red fairy grass of Jing Tian, it also became a fine herb that can ward off diseases and keep healthy.

天麻

有一年，大山深处的村子里突然流行起一种奇怪的疾病，发病时人们头痛得像裂开一样，严重时还会四肢抽搐，半身瘫痪。村里的乡亲到处求医问药，都不见效果。村里有个小伙子叫天生，他听说滴翠峡有个神医能治这种病，于是带了干粮，历经千辛万苦终于爬上神医所在的山顶，没想到天生突然感到头晕目眩，一头栽到地上，四肢抽搐，随后就什么也不知道了。醒来后，他发现自己睡在一间茅屋中，头也不痛了，四肢也不再抽搐。他起身打量茅屋里的东西，发现桌子上堆着一些像马铃薯一样的植物根茎。正在这时，从屋外走进来一位老人，手中端着一碗药，让天生喝下。老人告诉天生，他生的病和村里百姓的病一样，要靠一种药材医治。药材已准备好，就放在桌子上，让天生病好后带回村子。天生赶紧起身下床，向老人恭恭敬敬地叩头，感谢老人的救命之恩。为了纪念神医送药的恩情，乡亲们给这种药材取名为"天麻"，意为上天恩赐的专治半身麻痹的神药。

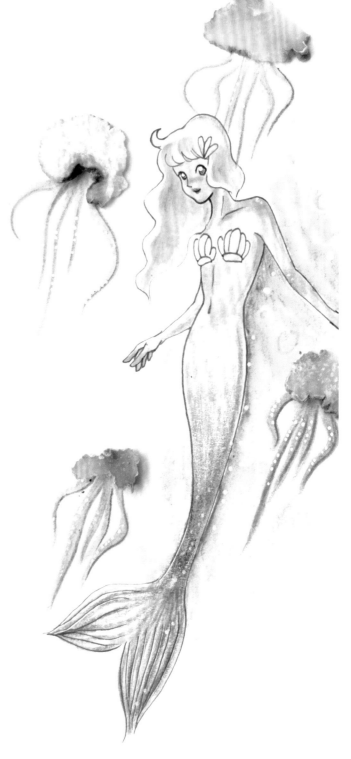

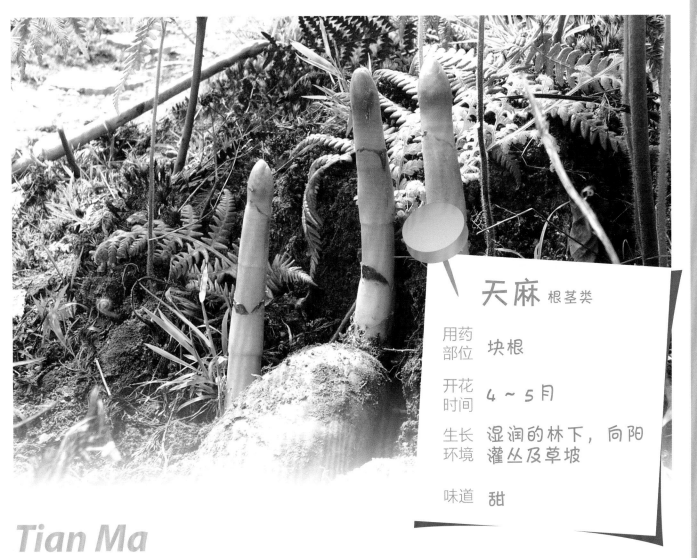

天麻 根茎类

用药部位	块根
开花时间	4～5月
生长环境	湿润的林下，向阳灌丛及草坡
味道	甜

Tian Ma

One year, a strange disease hit the village which was hidden deep in the mountains. It was present with splitting headache, convulsions and paralysis in severe conditions. The villagers sought medical advice everywhere, but nothing worked. A lad called Tian Sheng heard that there was an excellent physician in Di Cui Gorge that can cure the disease. Therefore, bringing some food with him, Tian Sheng went through difficulties and hardships to reach the top of the mountain. Unexpectedly, when he arrived at the top of the mountain, with dizziness, he threw himself on the ground. After convulsions, he lost his consciousness. When he woke up, he found himself in a hut with no pain in his head or limbs. After getting up, he looked around and found that there were some lumps of potato-like roots on the table. Just then, an old man came with a bowl of decection and asked Tian Sheng to drink it. The old man said that his illness was the same as the disease striking the village. There was a kind of herb that can treat it well. The herbs were ready on the table for being brought back to the village after Tian Sheng's recovery. Hearing this, Tian Sheng rose to his feet and kowtowed to the old man for his help. In order to commemorate the medicinal materials sent by the physician, they named the herb Tian Ma .(天麻 ; Tian means god and Ma refers to paralysis which mean it was a gift from the gods and it cured paralysis.)

太子参

春秋时期，郑国的王子年方五岁，天资聪慧，国王非常喜欢他。不幸的是，这位王子体质很差，常常生病，皇宫里的医生也对此束手无策，因此，国王通告天下求医问药，并许诺丰厚回报。有一天，一位白发老人来献药，说不是为了奖赏，而是为了医治好王子的病，让王子能够为国家百姓服务。国王对老者说："你有心了，可是如果药没有效果，可是欺君之罪。"老者笑道："王子身体稚嫩，难以承受强烈的补药，需慢慢补养。我有一种药物，服用一百天一定有效。"于是，王子按照方法服用老者所献的这种细长条状、黄白色的草根。三个月后，果然王子身体日益强壮。国王这才相信了老人所说的话，晋封王子为太子，又下令寻找老者，准备给他大大的奖励，却再也找不到老者踪迹了。国王问药物的名字，大家都摇头不知。有位大臣就说："药有参类的滋补作用，挽救太子的健康，就叫'太子参'吧。""太子参"的美名就这样传开了。

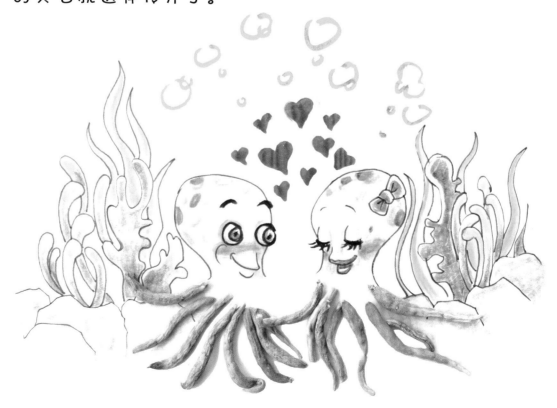

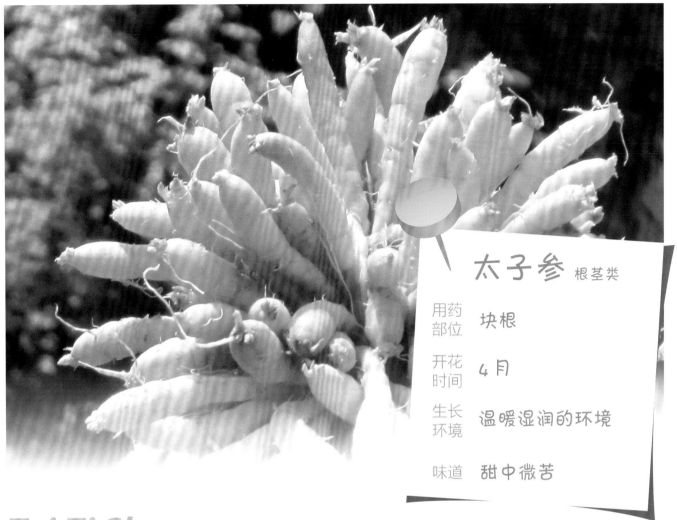

太子参 根茎类

用药部位	块根
开花时间	4月
生长环境	温暖湿润的环境
味道	甜中微苦

Tai Zi Shen

In the period of Spring and Autumn, the prince of Zheng State, though aged five, was gifted with wisdom. The king loved him very much, but with poor constitution, the prince frequently got sick, and the imperial physicians could do nothing about it. Therefore, the king put up an imperial notice to seek medical advice with promises of good returns. One day, a white-haired old man came to offer medicine, saying that he was not for the reward but for healing the prince's disease so that the prince could serve the people of the country. The king said to the old man: "Thank you for your kind heart, but if the medicine does not work, you'll commit the crime of deceiving the king." The old man smiled: "The prince is too young to take strong tonic herbs. I have a herb that will work if the prince takes it for one hundred days." So the prince took the long, thin, yellow-white grass roots offered by the old man. After three months, the prince got stronger. At this time, the king believed what the old man said and promoted the prince to crowned prince, and ordered the officials to find the old man in order to give him a reward. However, they could not find the old man. When the kings asked the name of the medicine, everyone shook their heads. One minister said: "The medicine has the tonic effects like ginseng, and it saved the crowned prince. Let's call it Tai Zi Shen (mans crowned prince ginseng)." the name of Tai Zi Shen was spread.

葛根

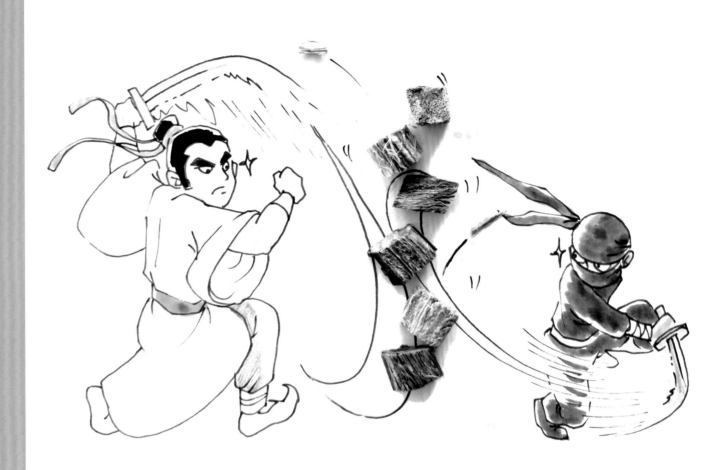

　　相传，山脚下住着一对年轻的夫妻，丈夫刻苦读书希望考取功名，妻子在家种田，照顾家庭。十年寒窗苦读之后，丈夫考中了进士。本来这是一件非常开心的事，可丈夫却非常烦恼。原来皇城里富家女子个个都丰盈美丽，而自己的妻子由于长年劳作，衰老瘦弱，于是就产生了和妻子离婚的念头。他托乡人带信回家，妻子打开只见两句诗"缘似落花如流水，驿道春风是牡丹"，妻子明白丈夫将要抛弃自己，终日茶饭不思，以泪洗面，容颜越发憔悴。山神得知后，怜爱善良苦命的女子，在梦中指引她每日上山挖食葛根。不久，妻子竟脱胎换骨，变得丰盈美丽，光彩照人。而丈夫托乡人送信后，思来想去觉得患难之妻不能抛弃。于是快马加鞭，赶回故里，发现妻子变得异常美貌，大喜过望，夫妻团圆，过上了美好生活。

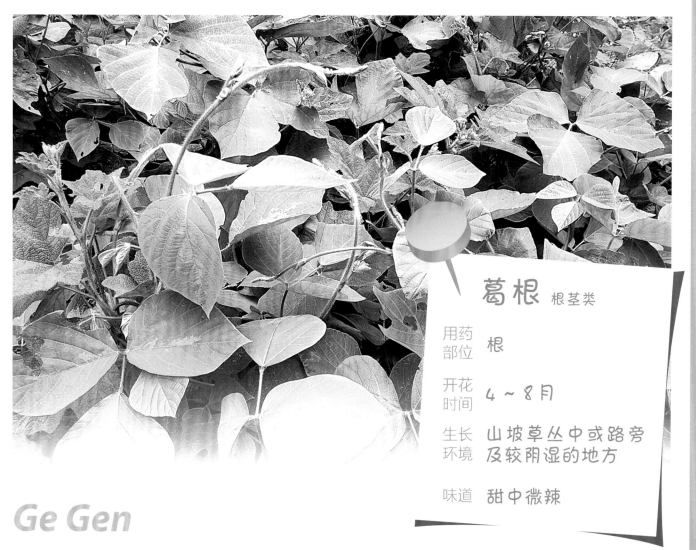

葛根 根茎类

用药部位	根
开花时间	4～8月
生长环境	山坡草丛中或路旁及较阴湿的地方
味道	甜中微辣

Ge Gen

   Legend has it that a young couple lived at the foot of a mountain. The husband studied hard and hoped to succeed in the imperial examination. The wife worked hard in the fields and took care of the family. After a decade of hard preparation, the husband passed the examination and became the candidate. It was a good thing, but the husband was very upset. He found that the girls in the imperial city were young, beautiful and rich, while his wife was thin, weak and old after years of hard work. With depression, he wanted to divorce his wife. He wrote a letter to his wife and asked the fellow villagers to take the letter home. The wife opened the letter and it was a poem that "fate flows away like a falling flower; the peony on the way is the true love." Knowing that the husband wanted to abandon her, the wife did nothing but cried all day. Therefore, she became weaker and weaker. When the mountain god heard of it, he pitied the kind and poor woman. Thus, he instructed the wife to dig for Ge Gen in the mountain every day in the dream. Soon, the wife changed greatly and became gorgeous. After sending the letter back home, the husband considered a lot and thought that how can he abandon the wife who was always there with him when he was in difficulty and hardship! So he hurried back home by riding horse. When he got home, he found that the wife became extremely beautiful. With great joy, the husband and the wife reunited and led a happy life ever since.

知母

一年冬天，一个老太婆蹒跚着来到一座偏远山村，身心憔悴，摔倒在一户人家门外。响声惊动了这家的主人。主人是个年轻樵夫，他把老人搀进屋里，嘘寒问暖，得知老人饿着肚子，急忙让妻子准备饭菜。樵夫夫妇对老人很好，把她当母亲一样看待，就这样过了三年多的幸福时光，老人到了八十岁的高龄。

这年夏天，她突然对樵夫说："孩子，你背我到山上看看吧。"樵夫不明就里，但还是愉快地答应了老人。他背着老人上坡下沟，跑东串西，累得汗流如雨，还不时和老人逗趣，老人始终很开心。他们来到一片野草丛生的山坡，老人下地，坐在一块石头上，指着一丛线型叶子、开有白中带紫条纹状花朵的野草说："把它的根挖来。"樵夫挖出一截黄褐色的草根，问："妈，这是什么？"老人说："这是一种药草，能治肺热咳嗽、身虚发烧之类的病，用途可大啦。孩子，你知道为什么直到今天我才教你认药么？"樵夫想了想说："妈妈是想找个老实厚道的人教他辨认药材的本领。怕居心不良的人拿这本事去发财，去坑害百姓！"老人点了点头

"孩子，你真懂得妈妈的心思。这种药还没有名字，你就叫它'知母'吧。"后来，老人又教樵夫认识了许多种药草。老人死后，樵夫改行采药，他一直牢记老人的话，真心实意为穷人送药治病。

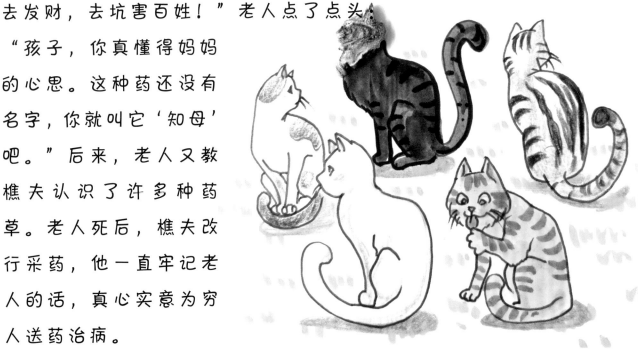

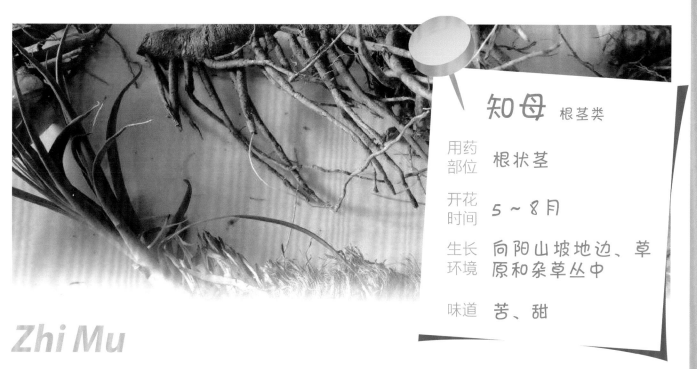

知母 根茎类

用药
部位 根状茎

开花
时间 5 ~ 8月

生长
环境 向阳山坡地边、草
原和杂草丛中

味道 苦、甜

Zhi Mu

One winter, an old woman lurched all the way to a remote village. Being worn out, the old woman collapsed in front of a house. The noise alarmed the house owner. The owner was a young woodcutter. He held the old woman into the house. Knowing the old woman was hungry, the woodcutter immediately asked his wife to cook. The young couple treated the old woman very well, regarded her as their mother. Three years later, the old woman turned 80 years old.

This summer, she suddenly said to the woodcutter, "My son, take me to the mountain." Although the woodcutter didn't understand the reason, he still agreed and carried the old woman up to the slope and down to the ditch, running east to the west. He was exhausted and sweated profusely. Even so, he occasionally told jokes to make the old woman laugh. When they came to a slope covered with weeds, the old woman got down and sat on a rock. Pointing to a clump of grasses with linear leaves and white flowers that were purple-striped in the middle of the petals, the old woman said: "Dig out their roots." The woodcutter dug out a yellow grass root and asked, "mom, what is this?" The old woman replied: "This is a kind of medicine. It can cure cough resulting from lung heat, fever due to weakness, and many other diseases. It's very useful. My boy, do you know why I didn't tell you the knowledge of medicine until today?" The woodcutter thought for a while and answered: "Because you want to teach the techniques to someone who is honest and kind. You are afraid that if the bad people know about it, they will make a fortune and do harms to people." The old woman nodded and said, "My son, you know what I am thinking about. This medicine has no name yet, let's call it Zhi Mu (literally means understanding mother)". Later, the old woman taught the woodcutter to know a lot of herbs. After the old woman died, the woodcutter became a herb picker and collector. Bearing what the old woman said in mind, he remained to be kind and always sent herbs to the poor.

党参

传说吕洞宾和铁拐李二位神仙从中原到太行山云游，看见四周犹如仙境一般，二仙赞叹不已。他们走到平顺地界时，忽然看见一头山猪在山坡上的土里乱拱，二仙童心未泯，想看个究竟，只见山猪拱过的地方，黑土疏松，油光发亮，土里长着一种类似豆秧的东西。铁拐李把它放在口中，边嚼边跟着吕洞宾赶路。走了很久，吕洞宾累得气喘吁吁，回头再看铁拐李，依然神情如常，紧紧跟随。

途中他们遇见一樵夫，樵夫说这种豆秧似的东西是一种神草。传说古时上党郡有户人家，每晚都隐约听到人的呼叫声，但每次出门看望，却始终不见其人。一天深夜，主人随声寻觅，终于在离家一里多远的地方，发现一株不平常的形体和人一样的植物，因出现在上党郡，所以叫"党参"。

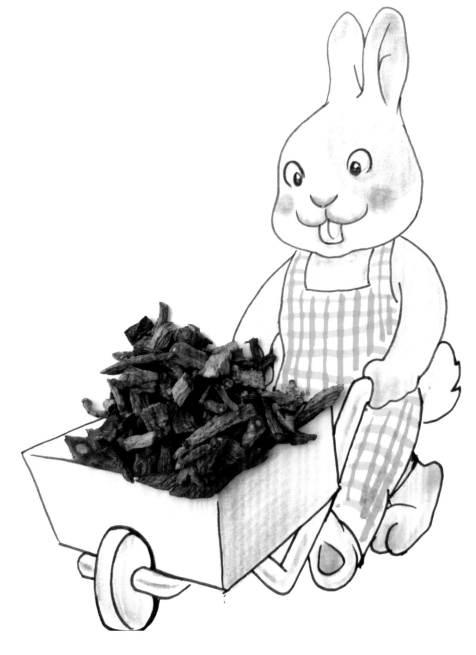

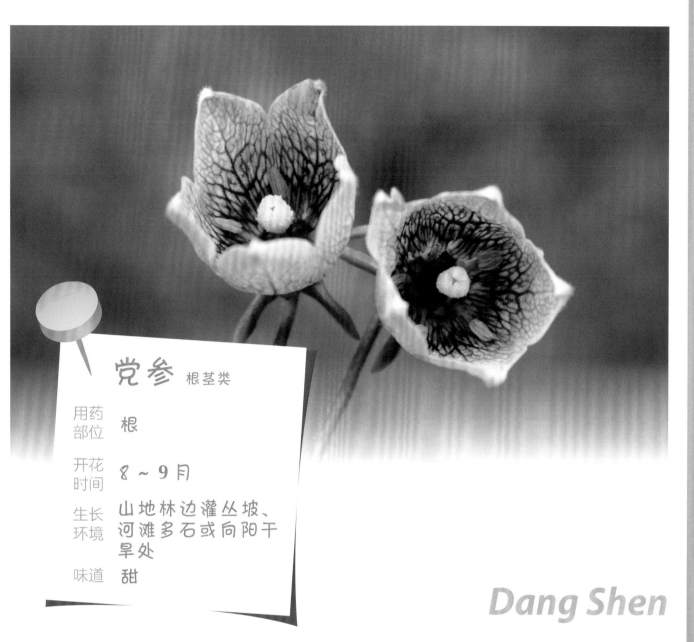

党参 根茎类

用药
部位 根

开花
时间 8～9月

生长
环境 山地林边灌丛坡、
河滩多石或向阳干
旱处

味道 甜

Dang Shen

It was said that when Lv Dongbin and Cripple Lee, two immortals, traveled from the Central Plains to Tai Hang Mountain, they were amazed at gorgeous scenery as if they were in a fairyland. When they walked to a plain, they suddenly saw a wild boar bumping against the hillside soils. Being curious, two immortals went over and found that the soil rushed by the boar was black, bright and loose and there grew something like soybean seedlings. Cripple Lee grabbed one, and chewed it while following Lv Dongbin. After a long walk, Lv Dongbin was exhausted and panted. Looking back, he found that Cripple Lee was so relaxed and closely followed.

On the way, they met a woodcutter. The woodcutter told them that what Cripple Lee took was a magic herb. It was said in ancient times, there was a family in Shang Dang prefacture who heard someone crying every night. They went out but found no one was there. One night, they followed the sound and at last found an unusual plant a mile away from home that looks like human being. As it was found in Shang Dang prefacture, so the herb was called Dang Shen.

玄参

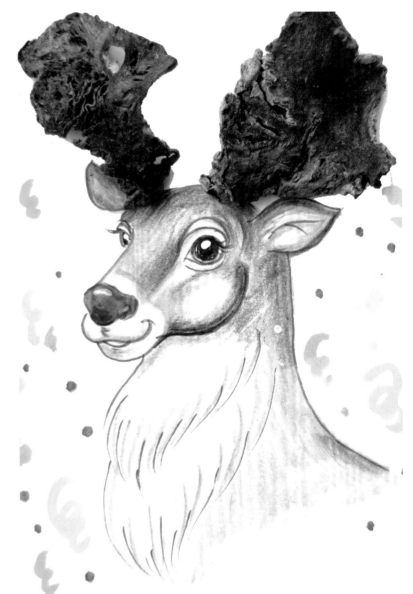

　　话说三国时期，蜀国大将张飞有一个特别的嗜好：一日三餐喜吃牛肉，还要大碗喝酒，酒后常常打骂自己的手下。其实，他打骂手下一是因为性格暴躁，还有一个更重要的原因就是张飞每天喝酒吃肉，以致内热伤阴，口腔常常如火上燎，牙痛起来真要命。于是，张飞吩咐手下拿钳子来，给他把牙拔掉，手下不敢，只得任其痛打。

　　一日，张飞的牙又痛起来，他挥舞着马鞭，不停地唤手下抱酒来。手下看张飞喝得太多，没有再去抱酒，结果被张飞的马鞭打得嗷嗷叫。另一个手下生性机灵，张飞一吩咐抱酒，就赶紧答应着去买。这个人从军前，在家里随爷爷学医。为了不被挨打，他在药铺买了半斤黑参，水煎成汤，倒进一些酒后端给了张飞。张飞醉意上涌，喝了一碗又一碗，还直叫道："好酒，好酒，快快再拿些来！"慢慢地，张飞不再发怒，牙也不痛了，酣然入梦。自那以后，手下一见张飞酒醉，就用黑参煎水当酒给他喝，张飞也不再因为牙痛而发脾气了（中药黑参，也就是现在所说的玄参）。

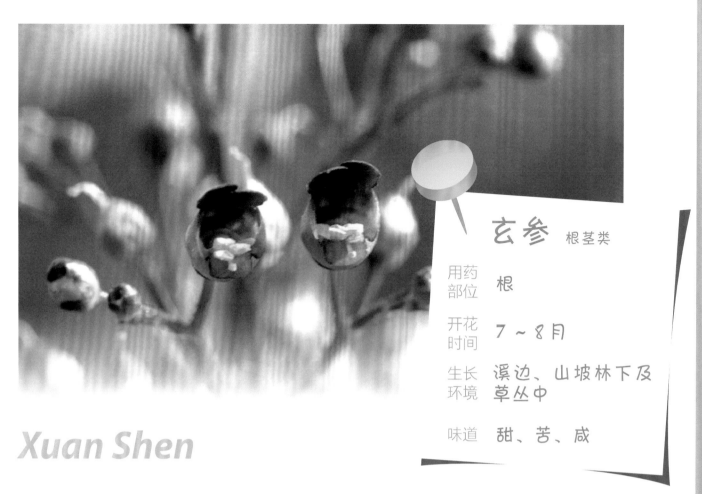

玄参 根茎类

用药部位	根
开花时间	7 ~ 8月
生长环境	溪边、山坡林下及草丛中
味道	甜、苦、咸

Xuan Shen

In the period of Three Kingdoms, Zhang Fei, the great general in Shu State had a special habit,he loved to eat beef and drink bowls of wine for three meals. After drinking, he often beat and scolded his soldiers. In fact, there were two reasons for his beating and scolding. One reason was his bad temper, the other reason and the more important one, was that his everyday intake of beef and wine caused internal heat harming the yin, resulting in scorching mouth. What made him more painful was the toothache that was killing him. So Zhang Fei ordered his men to take a clamp and to pull his teeth out. However, his men didn't dare to do it. So they had no choice but to be beaten.

One day, the toothache occurred again. So he waved a horse whip, and repeatedly called his men to serve wine. Seeing Zhang Fei had already drunk too much , they didn't serve wine. As a result, they were beaten again. There was one staff worker who was smart. Once Zhang Fei commanded him to serve wine, he immediately agreed to buy wine. Before joining in the army, this staff learned traditional Chinese medicine from his grandfather. In order not to be beaten, he bought half Jin (1 Jin=0.5 kilogram) of black ginseng from the herb shop and boiled it. Then he poured the decoction into the wine and served the mixed wine to Zhang Fei. Being drunk, Zhang Fei took a bowl of wine after another, and called to the staff ,"Good wine, give me more!" Gradually, Zhang Fei was no longer angry, and his teeth did not hurt. He slept well. Since then, once seeing Zhang Fei was drunk, the staff would boil black ginseng and mix it with wine. Zhang Fei never lost temper because of toothache. (The black ginseng in Chinese medicine is now called Xuan Shen.)

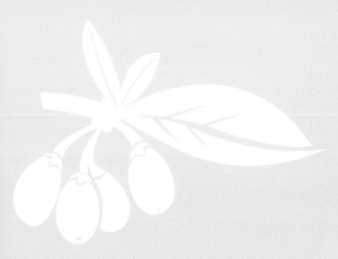

种子类
Seeds

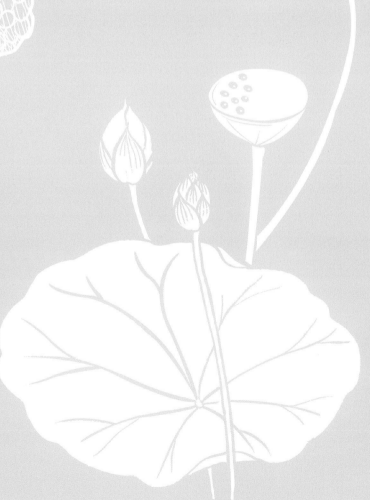

菟丝子

　　小山养了一只小兔子，活泼可爱，也很调皮。有一天小兔子在小明家院子里的草地上玩，不小心扭伤了腰，站不起来。小山很担心小兔子，一位路过的白胡子老爷爷看到了难过的小山，安慰他说："别担心，我有办法。"

　　老爷爷把受伤的小兔子放到一片黄豆地里。小山看到小兔子虽然身体不能动，却把脖子伸出来，吃豆秸上的一种藤蔓的种子。老爷爷让小明每天都来这里，让小兔子吃这种藤蔓的种子。慢慢地小兔子身体好了，又活蹦乱跳起来。

　　后来，小山采了这种小种子，分给有腰酸背痛症状的邻居们吃，邻居们吃了以后腰不酸背也不疼了。大家都很感激小山，问小山这种小种子叫什么名字，小山想起自己养的那只可爱的小兔子，就对大家说："叫它'菟丝子'吧"。

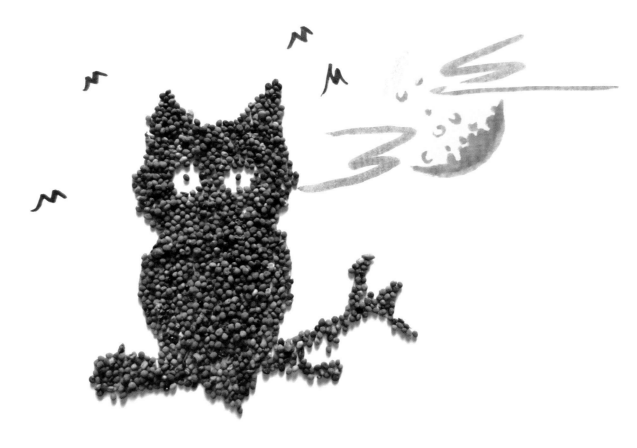

Tu Si Zi

The bunny raised by Xiao Shan was lovely but also naughty. One day, the bunny accidentally sprained its waist while playing on the yard and couldn't stand up. Xiao Shan was worried. The white-bearded old man,a passing by saw that Xiao Shan was very sad and comforted him: "Don't worry. I have come up with a solution"

The old man brought the injured bunny to the farmland of soybeans and put it on the ground. Xiao Shan noticed that the bunny, though unable to move, held out its neck and chewed the seed of a vine growing on the stalk. The old man asked Xiao Shan to bring the bunny here and feed it with the seeds every day. Gradually, the bunny got better and recovered.

Later, Xiao Shan picked up the small seeds and gave them to the neighbors who suffered from back pain. After the neighbors took them, they were not painful any more. They all appreciated Xiao Shan and asked him the name of the seeds. Thinking of the bunny he raised, he told everyone that the seeds was called "Tu Si Zi (Tu literally means bunny; Zi refers to seeds.)"

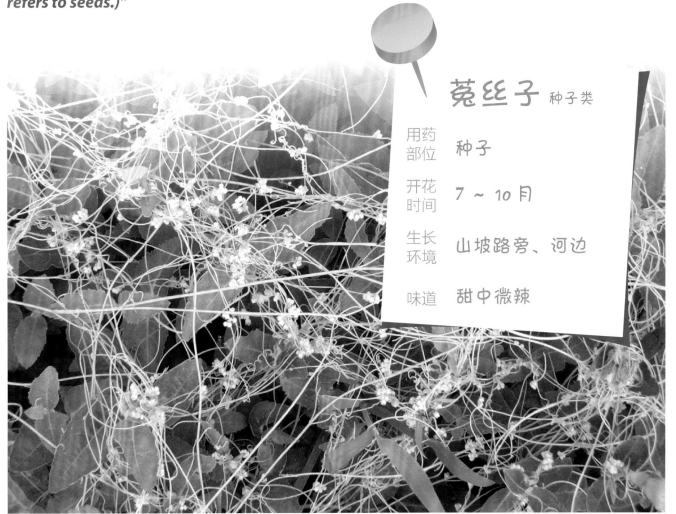

菟丝子 种子类

用药部位	种子
开花时间	7 ~ 10 月
生长环境	山坡路旁、河边
味道	甜中微辣

莱菔子

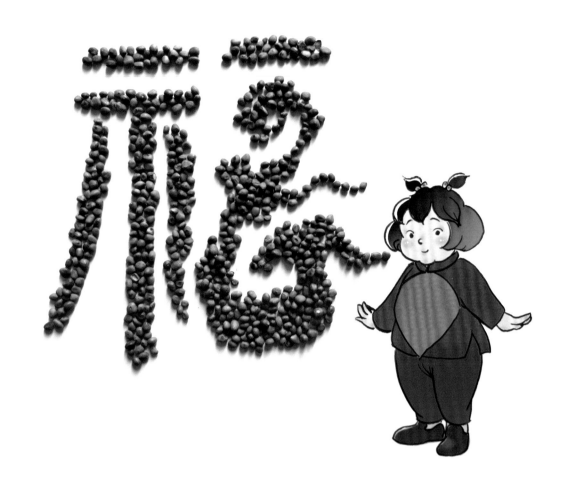

　　女皇武则天一直忙着国家大事，很辛苦。有一天她累坏了，躺在床上起不来。御医们急忙诊治，按照以前的方法在她吃的东西里加了很多补益的药材。女皇吃了药后觉得头晕眼花，不想吃东西，一生气就流鼻血。御医们吓坏了，却没有好的办法，最后一致同意贴出皇榜寻求帮助。

　　有个小医生见到告示，便揭下皇榜进宫为女皇看病。在给女皇诊脉后，他不慌不忙地从药袋里取出三钱萝卜籽，萝卜籽也叫"莱菔子"。小医生把它们研成粉末，做成三个丸子，让女皇吃。一丸吃下去，鼻血就止住了；二丸下去，头晕也好了；三丸吃光，女皇胃口大开，感觉自己已经完全恢复了。

　　女皇病好了，给了小医生很多的奖赏。

Wu Zetian, the empress in Tang dynasty, was very busy with the state affairs. One day, she was too exhausted to get up. The imperial physicians diagnosed and treated her. Following the previous therapeutic method, the physicians added a lot of nutritious herbs. However, the empress felt dizzy and had no appetite. Moreover, she suffered from nasal bleeding when she was angry. The imperial physicians were terrified. With no better treatment, they finally agreed to put up an imperial notice for seeking help.

When seeing the notice, a young physician took off the notice and entered the palace. After taking the pulse, he took out three qian (1 qian=5 grams) of the radish seeds in his pouch unhurriedly. This kind of radish seeds was called "Lai Fu Zi." The young physician ground the seeds into powder which made were into three pills for the empress. After taking one pill, the nasal bleeding was stopped; two pills, the dizziness was gone; three pills, she empress felt much better and had a great appetite.

The empress recovered and paid the young physician a lot.

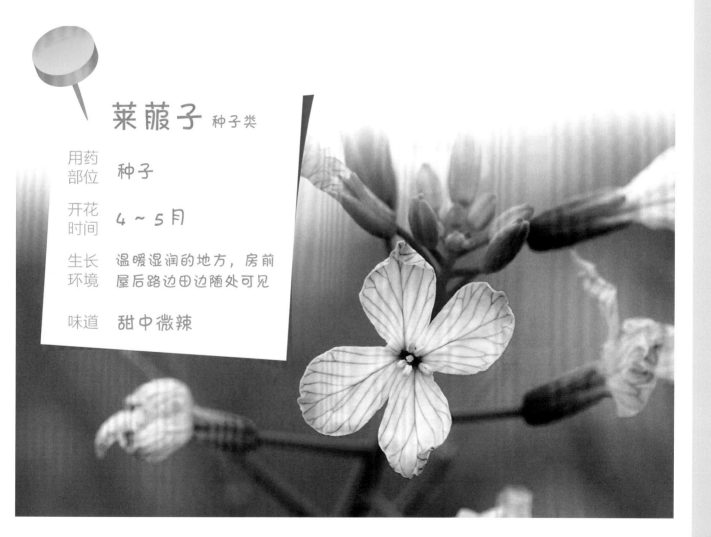

莱菔子 种子类

用药部位	种子
开花时间	4～5月
生长环境	温暖湿润的地方，房前屋后路边田边随处可见
味道	甜中微辣

王不留行

相传，西晋文学家左思成亲后不久，妻子便生下小宝宝惠芳。但是，妻子产后乳汁不通畅，小宝宝饿得哇哇直哭。左思夫妇心中十分着急，四处寻医，想要得到通畅乳汁的法子。一天，左思忽然听到一阵优美动听的乡土歌声："穿山甲、王不留，妇人服后乳长流……"左思循着歌声找去，看到唱歌的是一位乡间医生，便走过去向医生询问。医生解释说穿山甲和王不留行子是两味中药，是他家祖父留下来的通乳秘方，非常适合乳汁缺少的产妇。左思马上把医生请到家里为妻子配药，左夫人服后不久，果然奶水通了而且乳量很多，小宝宝自然也不用挨饿了。

后来，左思写下了王不留行治愈乳汁不下的诗句："产后乳少听吾言，山甲留行不用煎。研细为末甜酒服，畅通乳道如井泉。"

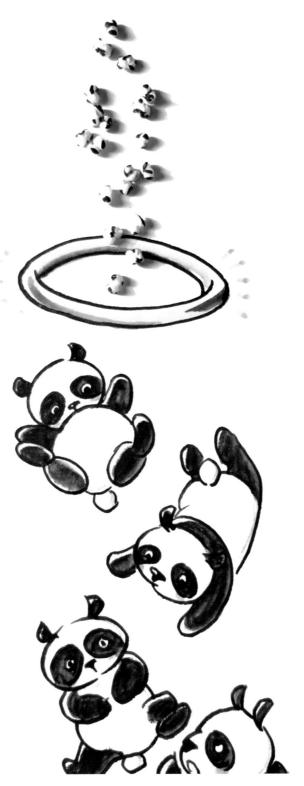

Wang Bu Liu Xing

Legend has it that Zuo Si, the litterateur in western Jin Dynasty, had a baby shortly after his wedding ceremony. However, his wife suffered from latex obstructead. The baby was starved and cried sadly. Zuo Si and his wife worried a lot. In an attempt to find a therapy for her problem, Zuo went out to seek physicians. Then he suddenly heard a beautiful song in a local accent, singing: "Milk flows freely after mothers take pangolins and cowherb seeds". Looking around hurriedly, Zuo found it was a local physician who sang the song. He went over and inquired about it. The physician explained that the pangolin and cowherb seeds, the two kinds of traditional Chinese medicine, were the secret recipes handed down from his grandfather. Both of them work very well for mothers with latex obstructed. Zuo Si immediately invited the physician to prescribe a therapy for his wife. Soon after taking the decoction, the milk flowed much more freely and the baby didn't starve again.

Therefore, Zuo Si wrote down the poem, appraising the cowherb seeds for promoting the lactation. The poem was that: "listen, the mother with scant milk, there was no need to boil pangolins and cowherb seeds. Grind them into powders and took them with sweet wine. The milk will flow freely like a spring."

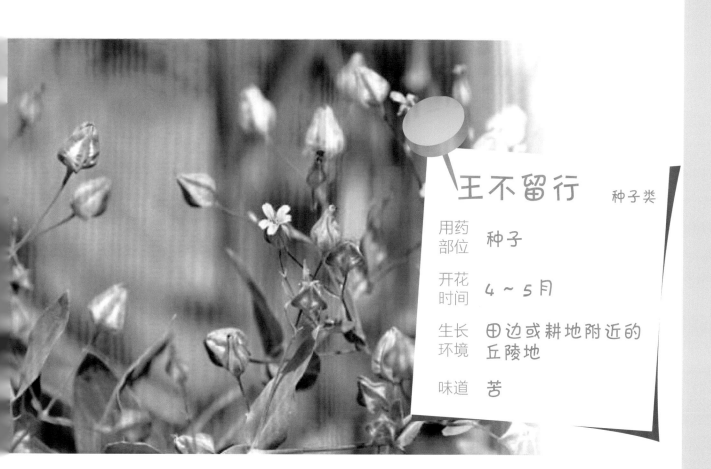

王不留行　种子类

用药部位	种子
开花时间	4～5月
生长环境	田边或耕地附近的丘陵地
味道	苦

薏苡仁

东汉时期，汉武帝派将军马援带兵与敌人交战。大军行进到一座深山老林，那里沼泽遍布，散发出毒气，天气早上很热，晚上又变得很冷，士兵们都觉得身体不适，浑身都湿湿的，渐渐失去了前进的力气，将军只好让士兵们停下来休息。

一天夜里，马援闷闷不乐地倚在帐篷里睡觉。忽然，一阵风吹过，有一位白发老人掀帘进来，这位老人手里拿着一株植物，上面结满像珍珠一样的果实，对马援说道："马将军一路辛苦了，这是薏苡仁，将军用水煮了让士兵们服用，可以让大伙恢复精神。"说完，老人就消失了。

第二天，马援醒来，立即派出军士进山搜寻这种植物，只见山谷下长满了薏苡仁。他非常高兴，让士兵们采摘回营煮着吃。没到两天，士兵们病证全消，士气大振。最终，马援带领士兵们打败了敌人，取得胜利。

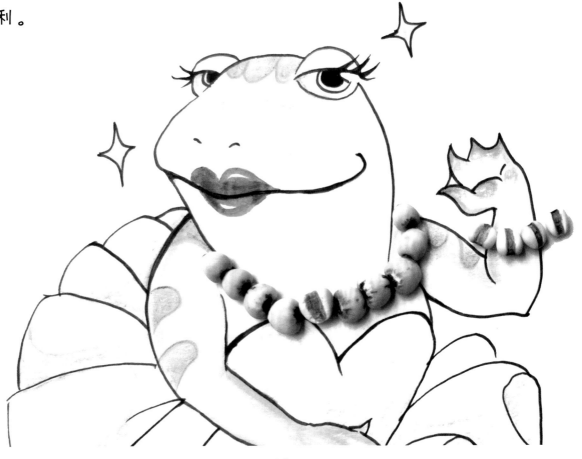

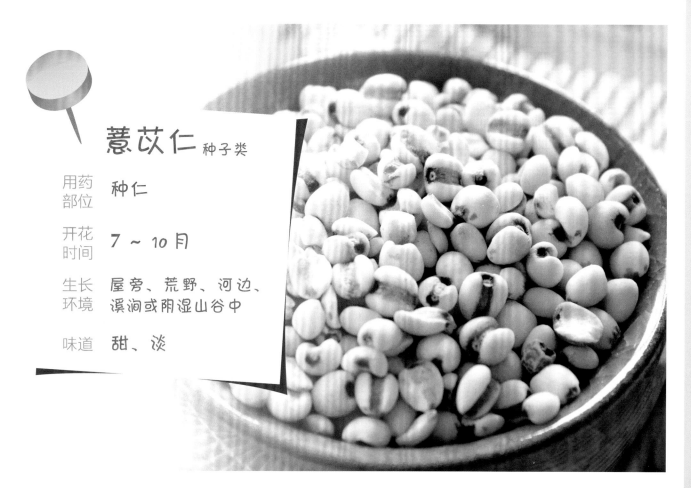

薏苡仁 种子类

用药部位	种仁
开花时间	7 ～ 10 月
生长环境	屋旁、荒野、河边、溪涧或阴湿山谷中
味道	甜、淡

Yi Yi Ren

In eastern Han Dynasty, Emperor Wu sent Ma Yuan, a general, to fight against the enemy. The army marched into a mountain where there were swamps, giving off poisonous gases. It was very hot in the morning and extremely cold in the evening. The soldiers felt damp and uncomfortable. Gradually, they lost the strength to advance, so the general had to let the soldiers have a rest.

One night, while the general was sleeping in his tent, a gust of wind blew and someone lifted the curtain and came in. It was a white-haired old man holding a plant full of pearl-like fruits. The old man said: "My general, you have marched so hard all the way. I'd like to send you these coix seeds. Boil them and drink the soup. They will refresh the soldiers." Then the old man disappeared.

The next day, after waking up, Ma Yuan immediately sent some soldiers into the mountain to search for this plant. The plant grew all over the valley. The general was enlightened. He told the soldiers to pick the seeds back and cooked them. Two days later, the soldiers felt better and the army had a better morale. Finally, the general led the soldiers and defeated the enemy.

白果

传说，很早以前有一位姓白的穷人家的姑娘，从小死了爹娘，12 岁就给财主放羊，受尽了人间苦难。一天，她在山坡上拾到了一枚奇异的果核，宝贝似地赏玩了几天还舍不得扔掉。最后把它种在了常去放羊的大刘山的一个山坳里。经过几年的精心照料，这颗神奇的种子生根发

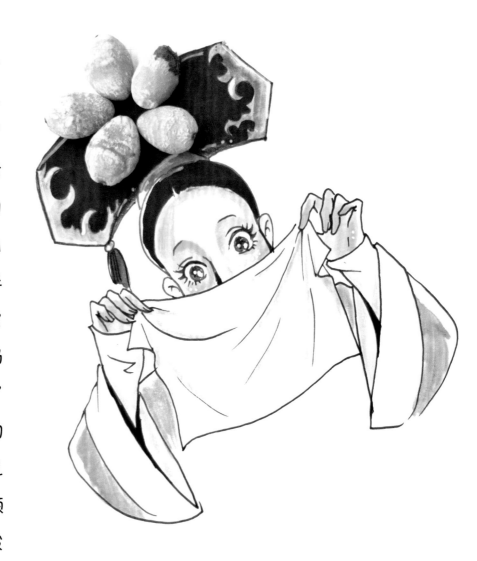

芽，长成了一棵参天大树，每年秋天都会结满黄澄澄的果子。一天白姑娘赶着羊群来到了这棵树下，突发咳嗽，痰涌咽喉吐咽不下，顿时昏迷过去。这时，从大树上飘下来一位美丽的仙女。手里拿着几颗从树上摘下的果子，取出果核，搓成碎末，一点一点地喂进白姑娘口中，片刻，白姑娘醒了。她慢慢睁开眼睛，仙女朝她笑了一下，飞上大树不见了。白姑娘赶紧从地上爬起来，从树上摘下许多果子，带到村里，送给有病的人吃，就这样治好了成千上万的咳喘病人。一传十，十传百，传来传去，人们干脆把"白姑娘送的果子"叫做白果，那结满白果的大树就叫做"白果树"了。也就是现在我们说的银杏树。

Bai Guo

It was said that long long ago, there was a poor girl. Her parents passed away when she was still young. At the age of 12, she began to herd sheep for landowners and suffered a lot. One day, she picked up a strange fruit kernel on the hillside and treasured it very much. Unwilling to throw it away, she planted it in a valley of Da Liu Mountain where she always herded sheep and took good care of it. Magically, the seed took root, sprouted and grew into a towering tree. Every autumn, the tree would bear yellow fruits. One day, the girl drove the sheep under the tree. With sudden coughs, the sputum surged into her throat. As she couldn't swallow it or spitted it up, she passed out. At this time, a beautiful fairy came down from the tree with some fruits. the fairy took out the kernels and grinded them into powder, then fed them to the girl. A moment later, the sputum stopped flowing upward and the girl opened her eyes. The fairy smiled at her and flew up to the tree and disappeared. The girl quickly got up from the ground, picked many fruits from the tree and brought them to the village for those who were sick. After taking the fruit, they all recovered. thousands of patients with coughing and asthma were cured. The story quickly spread from one person to another. The phrase "the fruit sent by the girl with the family of Bai (means white)" was shortened as the word "Bai Guo" (means white fruit), and the tree bearing Bai Guo was named "Bai Guo tree."

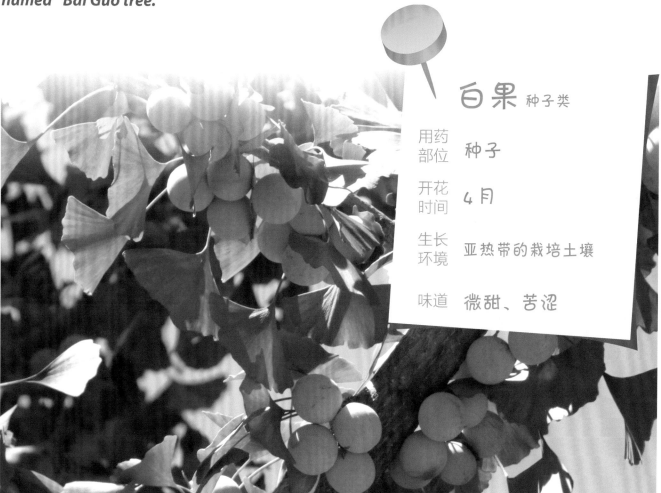

白果 种子类

用药部位	种子
开花时间	4月
生长环境	亚热带的栽培土壤
味道	微甜、苦涩

中医古籍
亲子阅读系列

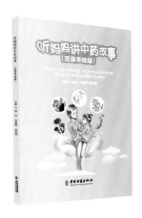

妈妈

    今天你还没给我讲故事呢

宝贝

    亲子阅读是我能为你做的最好的事

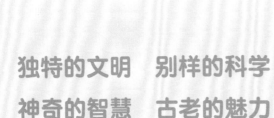

独特的文明　别样的科学

神奇的智慧　古老的魅力

孩子也能看懂的中医文化

中医药文化传承